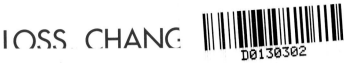

LOSS CHANG

D0130302

FACING DEATH

Series editor: David Clark, Professor of Medical Sociology,
University of Lancaster

The subject of death in late modern culture has become a rich field of theoretical, clinical and policy interest. Widely regarded as a taboo until recent times, death now engages a growing interest among social scientists, practitioners and those responsible for the organization and delivery of human services. Indeed, how we die has become a powerful commentary on how we live, and the specialized care of dying people holds an important place within modern health and social care.

This series captures such developments. Among the contributors are leading experts in death studies, from sociology, anthropology, social psychology, ethics, nursing, medicine and pastoral care. A particular feature of the series is its attention to the developing field of palliative care, viewed from the perspectives of practitioners, planners and policy analysts; here several authors adopt a multidisciplinary approach, drawing on recent research, policy and organizational commentary, and reviews of evidence-based practice. Written in a clear, accessible style, the entire series will be essential reading for students of death, dying and bereavement, and for anyone with an involvement in palliative care research, service delivery or policy-making.

Current and forthcoming titles:

David Clark, Jo Hockley and Sam Ahmedzai (eds): *New Themes in Palliative Care*
David Clark and Jane E. Seymour: *Reflections on Palliative Care*
David Clark and Michael Wright: *Transitions in End of Life Care: Hospice and Related Developments in Eastern Europe and Central Asia*
Mark Cobb: *The Dying Soul: Spiritual Care at the End of Life*
Kirsten Costain Schou and Jenny Hewison: *Experiencing Cancer: Quality of Life in Treatment*
David Field, David Clark, Jessica Corner and Carol Davis (eds): *Researching Palliative Care*
Pam Firth, Gill Luff and David Oliviere: *Loss, Change and Bereavement in Palliative Care*
Anne Grinyer: *Cancer in Young Adults: Through Parents' Eyes*
Henk ten Have and David Clark (eds): *The Ethics of Palliative Care: European Perspectives*
Jenny Hockey, Jeanne Katz and Neil Small (eds): *Grief, Mourning and Death Ritual*
Jo Hockley and David Clark (eds): *Palliative Care for Older People in Care Homes*
David W. Kissane and Sidney Bloch: *Family Focused Grief Therapy*
Gordon Riches and Pam Dawson: *An Intimate Loneliness: Supporting Bereaved Parents and Siblings*
Lars Sandman: *A Good Death: On the Value of Death and Dying*
Jane E. Seymour: *Critical Moments: Death and Dying in Intensive Care*
Anne-Mei The: *Palliative Care and Communication: Experiences in the Clinic*
Tony Walter: *On Bereavement: The Culture of Grief*
Simon Woods: *Death's Dominion: Ethics at the End of Life*

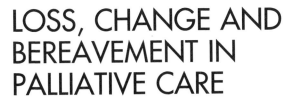

LOSS, CHANGE AND BEREAVEMENT IN PALLIATIVE CARE

PAM FIRTH
GILL LUFF
and DAVID OLIVIERE

OPEN UNIVERSITY PRESS

Open University Press
McGraw-Hill Education
McGraw-Hill House
Shoppenhangers Road
Maidenhead
Berkshire
England
SL6 2QL

email: enquiries@openup.co.uk
world wide web: www.openup.co.uk

and Two Penn Plaza, New York, NY 10121–2289, USA

First published 2005

A catalogue record of this book is available from the British Library

ISBN 0 335 21323 5 (pb) 0 335 21324 3 (hb)

Library of Congress Cataloging-in-Publication Data
CIP data applied for

Typeset by YHT Ltd, London
Printed in Great Britain by MPG Books Ltd, Bodmin, Cornwall

Contents

Notes on the contributors

Lesley Adshead currently combines research and teaching in palliative care with a research post in a medical school. She has many years experience working in advice and social work settings, including working as Senior Welfare Rights Officer for people with HIV/AIDS at a London hospital, and as a specialist palliative care social worker at St John's Hospice, London.

Jenny Altschuler is a clinical psychologist and family psychotherapist, working as a freelance consultant to professionals in health care settings, and Psychotherapy Consultant and Trainer for a Kosovo-based project for families affected by war – the One to One Family Centres. She is also currently working as a researcher at The Open University. Jenny is the author of *Working with Chronic Illness* (Macmillan, 1997).

Peter Beresford is Professor of Social Policy and Director of the Centre for Citizen Participation at Brunel University, and a Visiting Fellow of the School of Social Work and Psychosocial Studies at the University of East Anglia. He is chair of Shaping Our Lives, the independent national user-controlled organization core funded by the Department of Health, and a Trustee of the Social Care Institute for Excellence.

Grace H. Christ, DSW, is an Associate Professor at Columbia University School of Social Work in New York City. She is currently the Director of the Social Work Council on Palliative and End-of-life Care, sponsored by the Project on Death in America, and director of the Fire Department of New York's post 11 September 2001 Family Assessment and Guidance programme. She was formerly Director of Social Work at Memorial Sloan-Kettering Cancer Center in New York City. Among other publications she is the author of *Healing Children's Grief* (Oxford University Press, 2000).

Suzy Croft is Senior Social Worker at St John's Hospice, London. She is a Trustee of Help the Hospices and Chair of the Association of Hospice and Specialist Palliative Care Social Workers. She is a member of the Editorial Collective of Critical Social Policy.

Pam Firth is Head of Family Support at Isabel Hospice, Welwyn Garden City, and freelance group worker and trainer. She previously worked in child and family psychiatric settings as a social worker and has lectured in social work at several universities. Pam is currently a UK Director of the European Association of Palliative Care and adviser to the Childhood Bereavement Network. She has written several articles and book chapters on childhood bereavement, groupwork and multi-professional teamwork.

Shirley Firth works as a freelance writer, lecturer and workshop leader on multicultural approaches to health, death, dying and bereavement. She has taught at Surrey and Reading Universities, as well as the Open University in the UK and at the University of Maine in the USA. Her most recent book is *Wider Horizons: Care of the Dying in a Multicultural Society* (NCHSPCS, 2001).

Richard Harding is Research Fellow in the Department of Palliative Care and Policy, Guy's, King's and St Thomas' School of Medicine, London. His areas of research and publication are in palliative care in Africa, HIV/AIDS palliative care, and group work and behavioural interventions.

Felicity Hearn is currently employed as senior trainer with the NHS Expert Patients Programme. She has previously worked as a specialist palliative care social worker and was involved in the development of the UK National Network for the Palliative Care of People with Learning Disabilities.

Jennie Lester is an experienced hospice social worker currently working as a freelance trainer in palliative care. Jennie's work on the concept of a structured life review with the terminally ill is the first systematic life review in palliative care in the UK. She has presented her work at a number of national and international conferences, and has made regular contributions on this subject for students on the MSc in Professional Studies in Palliative Care.

Gill Luff is an independent consultant in palliative care, working with major cancer charities to develop educational projects and staff support. She set up the social work and bereavement service at St Peter's Hospice, Bristol, UK where she worked for a decade. As Macmillan Senior Lecturer in Palliative Care Social Work at the University of Gloucestershire, Gill developed multi-professional palliative care education, and chaired the Association of Hospice and Specialist Palliative Care Social Workers. She is currently a member of the steering committee of the Bereavement Research Forum.

Linda Machin is an Honorary Research Fellow at Keele University, UK, and does freelance training and hospice counselling. Linda began her career as a medical social worker. She was a founder member of the national Bereavement Research Forum and was its Chair for three years. Linda also initiated one of the first certificate courses in Bereavement Studies in the UK. Her publications include: *Working with Young People in Loss Situations* (Longman, 1993), *Looking at Loss* (Pavilion, 1990) and 'Women's voices in bereavement' in M. Bernard, J. Phillips, L. Machin and V.H. Davies, *Women Ageing* (Routledge, 2000).

Jan McLaren is the inaugural Director of the Laura Centre, a bereavement counselling centre in Leicester, UK. She was a research fellow at the Institute of Medical Sociology in Aberdeen for eleven years, and after retraining as a person-centred counsellor and psychotherapist, was the first manager of ACIS, a community counselling centre in Aberdeen. She is currently undertaking research into the effects of the death of a child upon bereaved parents.

David Oliviere is Director of Education and Training, St Christopher's Hospice, and Visiting Professor, School of Health and Social Sciences, Middlesex University, UK. With a background in psychiatric social work and management in the personal social services, David was involved with Pilgrim's Hospice, Canterbury, before joining the North London Hospice as Director of Social Work. Subsequently, David worked as Community Care Advisor for ethnic minorities and refugees in London, and more recently as Macmillan Principal Lecturer in Palliative Care at Middlesex University, whilst practising at the Macmillan Support Team at Barnet Hospital. He has written a number of chapters, articles and books on palliative care. The most recent jointly edited with Barbara Monroe, *Patient Participation in Palliative Care: A Voice for the Voiceless* (Oxford University Press, 2003) and *Death, Dying and Social Differences* (Oxford University Press, 2004).

Ann Quinn is Director of Social Work Studies within the School of Health and Social Care at Reading University. She qualified as a social worker in Australia, but has worked in the UK since 1976, in a variety of social care settings, including hospice work. Recent publications include: *Macmillan Cancer Relief Study into Benefits Advice for People with Cancer* (Macmillan Cancer Relief, 2002) and A. Quinn, A. Snowling and P. Denicolo, *Older People's Perspectives: Devising Information, Advice and Advocacy Services* (Joseph Rowntree Foundation, 2003). Her website is at www.rdg.ac.uk/health/staff/quinn.html

Phyllis R. Silverman is a Scholar-in-Residence at the Women's Studies Research Center at Brandeis University, and Associate in Social Welfare at Massachusetts General Hospital, Harvard Medical School, USA. Her publications include: the co-edited *Continuing Bonds: A New*

Understanding of Grief, Never Too Young to Know: Death in Children's Lives, and a new edition of *Widow-to-Widow*. In addition, Phyllis has co-edited a new resource for end-of-life care entitled *Living with Dying*. Her website provides more information about her work: www.phyllisrsilver man.com

Jean Walker identifies as a user of palliative care services in the UK. She is actively involved as a service user both locally and nationally. She is a member of the User Involvement Panel established by Help the Hospices and the National Council for Hospice and Specialist Palliative Care Services.

Karen Wilman identifies as a user of palliative care services in the UK. She is actively involved as a service user both locally and nationally. She is a member of the User Involvement Panel established by Help the Hospices and the National Council for Hospice and Specialist Palliative Care Services.

Series editor's preface

In the spring of 1993 my father suffered an aortic aneurism and was admitted to hospital for emergency surgery. On hearing the news I left my office at the university and drove north about 100 miles to be with my mother as quickly as I could. I am the youngest of three and my two older brothers were both outside the country, one living in Portugal, the other on holiday in France. On the first evening my mother and I were shocked at the turn of events, but imbued with plenty of fighting spirit that my father would pull though the surgery and make some sort of recovery. I pushed away thoughts about his declining trajectory in the months prior and tried not to think too hard about what his future quality of life might be like.

Around midnight we were admitted to the intensive care unit where my father had been taken after his operation. I remember being surprised by the noise of the machines and the brightness of the lights. We stayed awhile at the bedside trying to take in the details of his situation and where it might be leading

Returning the following morning, we began to learn the routines that would shape my father's care in the coming days: the technical monitoring, the constant attention, and the respectful and caring way in which the nurses looked after their unconscious patient. My brothers arrived from distant places, we stayed at the family home and with my mother at the centre of things, we shared in a daily bedside presence. I got to know and to like the staff in the intensive care unit, though my question about whether we would move to palliative care at some point received a rather blank response. One day when I had returned home to my own young family and to deal with things at work, my father regained consciousness and was briefly weaned off the ventilator. It was a precious moment for my mother and my two brothers.

Thereafter, things became more complicated. Renal problems began to develop. At the end of the first week a decision had to be taken to move my father to a dialysis unit in another hospital about five miles away. A positive rationale was given and on arrival, the consultant talked about similar patients to my father who had 'walked out' of his unit.

In fact things quickly worsened. A few evenings later, we all gathered in the noisy and impersonal cubicle, uncertain whether our father was alive or dead, grieving and unsure what was going to happen next. There seemed to be no plan among the staff about how to (as Cicely Saunders might put it) 'gather up' the whole situation. I asked if it was time to switch off the ventilator and was told by a nurse that this was not hospital policy. A few minutes later we were all asked to leave for a while to facilitate a shift handover. We went to sit quietly in the hospital chapel. After half an hour, one of my brother's and I returned to the unit. As we walked in a nurse rushed towards us and announced that 'your father has in fact died'. I asked to see him and spent a few moments there in the messy aftermath. We returned and broke the news to our mother. I am sure each one of us felt that we had failed to be with our father at the moment of his death.

Later as we left the hospital we met with the consultant, coming into the building. He looked uncomfortable and with no other words of introduction told us; 'remember him as he was, not how he has been here'. As both a form of condolence and as a guide to future action, his words were hopelessly inadequate. We came away, arranged the funeral, said farewell to our father and got on with the rest of our lives. We had no further contact with any of the staff who had cared for my father, though I did return to both hospitals on occasions to visit other relatives being cared for there.

For years afterwards I felt bad about my father's death. I spoke about it only briefly with my mother and brothers and instead threw my energy into my palliative care research. I came to understand that death in the hospital, as Friedmann Nauck once told me, is often like an 'industrial accident'- a situation which is treated as if it is unexpected, occurring for the first time, and in an ideal world would be avoidable. I have learned to live with my grief, my loss and the changes they have brought to my life.

And that is where the connection with the present volume occurs. Pam Firth, Gill Luff, David Oliviere and all the other contributors to this book care deeply about the culture and social organisation of death, dying and bereavement in our society. Together they have produced a set of writings that explore these issues in the palliative care context. Their book builds on and adds to other contributions to the *Facing Death* series. It is an admirable complement to the collection edited by Jenny Hockey and colleagues (2001) on *Grief, Mourning and Death Ritual*; it resonates with and picks up some of the themes to be found in Tony Walter's (1999) *On Bereavement*; and it shares some of the perspectives found in Gordon Riches and Pam Dawson's (2000) *An Intimate Loneliness*. This is the seventeenth volume in the *Facing Death* series. I congratulate the editors on its production and commend their book to anyone concerned about how social and organisational forces shape the manner of our dying in the modern world – and what can be done about it.

David Clark

References

Hockey, J Katz, J and Small, N eds (2001) *Grief, Mourning and Death Ritual*. Buckingham: Open University Press.

Walter, T (1999) *On Bereavement*. Buckingham: Open University Press.

G Riches and P Dawson (2000) *An Intimate Loneliness*. Buckingham: Open University Press.

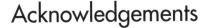

Acknowledgements

An edited book is the culmination of the work of many. Our grateful thanks go to all the authors who have generously contributed their experience and have worked for the benefit of others. To Professor David Clark for the opportunity to be part of his Facing Death series and for his helpful comments in the planning and on the final draft.

To Barbara Monroe for her support and Foreword and her leadership in palliative care. To Jacinta Evans, in the early stages, and to Rachel Gear of Open University Press for their help and guidance. To Annamaria Di Stefano at Isabel Hospice for her excellent and consistent administrative support.

A special mention to our friend and colleague of many years, the late Frances Sheldon, pioneer of psychosocial palliative care, fellow social worker and Macmillan Lecturer. Frances's integrity was an anchor to us and to many who knew her and her work in the field of multi-professional palliative care. She was a great advocate for patients, clients, families and communities, and influenced a whole generation of students.

Finally to our partners and children for putting up with years of 'loss, change and bereavement', as our enthusiasm frequently worked overtime, and for constantly hearing about death and bereavement. Our thanks to them all for their sense of humour, patience and support in our explorations into how people can be transformed by their experiences of loss.

Pam Firth
Gill Luff
David Oliviere

Foreword

This book offers a rich mix of chapters that together provide a commentary on current themes and developments surrounding loss, change and bereavement in palliative care, and a reminder of the value of integrating theory, research, practice and service development. The volume provides useful updates in a number of key areas, for example user involvement, carers, the forces of exclusion, the challenges of changing demographics and appropriate responses to diversity. It charts clearly the shifting emphasis from an individual, often medicalized model of loss, to one that places the individual firmly in a family, social and cultural context and acknowledges that the values and attitudes of society (including those of professional helpers) affect the ways in which people grieve. Structural inequalities can increase disadvantage and vulnerability; palliative care should include a recognition of the importance of the political dimension and a willingness to act upon it.

The importance of narrative emerges as a strong theme. These stories of explanation and meaning can represent both individual and self-defined constructions, and powerful external impositions upon the individual by dominant agencies including community groups, families and organizations. Narratives can support and encourage coping but may also pinion and limit the options of the individual facing loss. There are challenges here for those of us involved in delivering palliative care, to return to its founding roots of listening, open enquiry and creative response. Is the current emphasis on an evidence-based approach helping us to respond to and to measure aspects of care important to particular individuals and communities, or to deliver to predetermined professional agendas?

Many recent requirements in end-of-life care (a pertinent example being the National Institute for Clinical Excellence's *Guidance on Improving*

Supportive and Palliative Care for Adults with Cancer (2004)) emphasize assessment of risk of health problems within individuals and the delineation of specific professional competences appropriate to each level of supposed need. Such responses are important as we seek equity of provision and delivery in a necessarily resource-constrained health care environment. They carry, however, the danger that we will lose the important focus in quality palliative care on possibilities as well as problems. Increasing interest is being devoted to the concept of resilience, to an examination of what helps individuals and groups to survive and thrive in the face of difficult or tragic life events, looking at protective as well as risk factors. This book encourages this important and welcome direction.

Specialist palliative care has developed high standards of service for people with cancer and is considering its response to other life-threatening illnesses. In the next decades an increasing number of people will live longer with life-threatening disease. Professional care cannot expand to meet this need on its own. Palliative care must also seek to support and work in partnership with the communities in which people live and to potentiate their understanding and skills in responding to dying and bereavement. We need a framework that focuses on developing hope and creativity as well as delivering bad news in an effective and risk-limiting manner. We need to interweave a wide range of professional health and social care responses with those of the community in a complex network of public and voluntary services, if we are to respond appropriately to the needs of individuals in a way that increases both their own resilience and that of the communities around them.

This book affirms that loss is everyone's business. Everyone will die, we will all experience bereavement. Dying, death and bereavement are social experiences in which the individual is profoundly affected by the responses of those around him. In the shifting strands that represent our current conceptions of loss it can seem that little is certain amidst the increasing complexities, that there is so much that we do not know. Some things remain clear: loss hurts, and we will all seek to manage this in different ways and use different supports to do so. Palliative care is challenged to respond creatively to this diversity.

Barbara Monroe
St Christopher's Hospice

Introduction

Pam Firth, Gill Luff and David Oliviere

Erica and Rick

Erica, in her sixties, with advanced ovarian cancer, entered a hospice for end-of-life care. Loss, change and bereavement were not foreign to her. What of Erica's background in understanding her care in the hospice and the past working in the present? Erica was completely blind and so was her husband, Rick. They had no children.

Erica arrived in the UK a 12-year-old Jewish girl from Austria at the outbreak of the Second World War, sent by her parents, not on the Kinderstransport but on transport organized by the Jewish Blind Society. Her parents planned to follow but never arrived. Erica arrived with a placard around her neck giving her name and the language she spoke. Not a word of English.

She was brought up in a residential school for the blind, was a very bright student and wanted to go to university and train as a social worker. However, she was discouraged from doing this. Nevertheless, she studied modern languages at the London School of Economics, including a year at the Sorbonne in Paris. Just prior to admission to the hospice, Erica was head of modern languages in a secondary school.

Transferred from hospital to the hospice, Erica had laid out all her things over her bed to manage her environment but the next day a member of staff entered her room and told Erica, 'We mustn't have things on the bed; when visitors come in, it looks bad.' The staff member tidied up Erica's possessions onto her bedside locker, without explaining to her where each thing was.

Erica was upset and remained 'thrown' by this incident for the three-week stay at the hospice before she died. She did not feel cared for or in control. Rick was grateful for the medical treatment but not impressed by the care given, and Erica died unhappy.

Rick continued to be troubled by his wife's distress. In his words, 'she had felt ignored and excluded'. Some weeks later, he went to see the nursing director and was told (or at least that was his understanding) that Erica was an angry person and that it was natural for him, too, to be angry in bereavement. To date, Rick ruminates on this incident and it remains a distinct feature in his bereavement.

A textbook putting language around loss, change and bereavement almost denies the depth and complexity of an *experience* that can touch every fibre of body, mind and spirit. Any attempt to explain these phenomena fails to do justice to the nature of bereavement and its physical, psychological, spiritual and social interplay.

The above remains one couple's narrative but it informs our search and research into best and inclusive bereavement support in palliative care. Erica and Rick's story challenges us to integrate our understanding and competence of multiple facets of loss, user feedback and involvement, change and bereavement service. In the palliative care community, we need to be open to the needs that Erica and Rick represent: their personal histories; the integration of professional and service user perspectives; and the importance of effective multi-professional teamwork in interventions before and after the death.

Hospices and palliative care services are not perfect, but we may hope that Erica and Rick's story is exceptional. However, palliative care cannot remain complacent about standards of care in responding to the experience of loss, change and bereavement and its manifestation in patients and their carers.

The research community needs to be critical about how the voice of the bereaved person is captured. Service provision needs to guard against depersonalization, discrimination and organizational domination as illustrated in this scenario. Audit, governance and complaints mechanisms need to be more personalized and time-giving in order to appreciate and meet the needs of a diverse public and users, including minorities. There are obvious implications for staff training by involving service users in the training process and acting on their feedback about service provision.

Decades after the initial work of the pioneers of palliative care, health and social care professionals are still pushing out the boundaries of understanding of loss, change and bereavement. Almost forty years since the founding of modern palliative care, professionals, volunteers and, increasingly, bereaved people themselves are discovering and extending our knowledge, theories and models of grief and bereavement.

This book builds on the vast literature already available on bereavement and advances our knowledge base in the areas of: research and theories;

work with bereaved children, parents, families and adults; the disadvantaged bereaved; the involvement of the users of services; responses to diversity; and specific approaches such as life story and groupwork. It presents an international perspective to many of these aspects as well as latest thinking, from the lessons learned from the 11 September 2001 disaster to the development of new ways of assessing and integrating phase/stage and dual process models of bereavement.

The book is firmly rooted in the psychosocial aspects of palliative care, with many of the contributors coming from the field of professional social work, counselling and family therapy together with academic and practitioner researchers, from the UK and the USA. The social and cultural context of people's lives is increasingly recognized as having great importance as people search for meaning in the face of loss and change. (Field 2000; Sheldon 2003). With growing interest in postgraduate studies in bereavement and palliative care around the world, we aim to provide an advanced textbook to be used by the expanding multi-professional audience, including those working in the wider field of health and social care.

Overview of the chapters

Ann Quinn, in the opening chapter, describes the past decade as a time of re-examination of older dominant models of grief and loss. The revolutionary aspect of new theories and models is emphasized: the way in which bereaved people's voices are heard and contribute to the current challenges to long-held beliefs and assumptions. The context that she examines relates mainly to the UK but she acknowledges the importance of international perspectives and developments amidst a growing awareness of individual and cultural diversity. She examines the development of specialist palliative care and draws attention to the variability of service provision for ill and bereaved people.

Phyllis R. Silverman provides a fuller critique of the models of loss and grief in western society using a social constructivist perspective in Chapter 2. She highlights how the values and attitudes of society affect the way in which people grieve. Until the twentieth century, religious faith and ritual helped people give expression and direction to their grief. Currently we observe bereaved people searching for other ways to find self-expression or to make sense of their loss. She concludes that grief is a universal experience and change is seen as an integral part of the grieving process, as well as drawing our attention to the fact that death ends a life and not a relationship.

Practioner research comes to the fore in Chapter 3 where Linda Machin concludes that listening to individual stories of grief helps us to learn new ways of looking at loss and bereavement and provides the opportunity to test the validity of existing theories. She examines three differing ways of responding to loss based on her own practice with adult bereaved people and the work of earlier attachment theorists.

Jenny Altschuler leads the reader to consider the impact of loss on the individual and his/her family in Chapter 4. She uses ideas from family therapy and systems theory to explore how adults and children adjust to the diagnosis of life threatening illness to a family member. She emphasizes the move away from research that focuses on risk factors, towards concepts such as resilience, and the mechanisms that reduce the negative chain reactions following the diagnosis of serious illness. Her definition of the family highlights the changes in family life in the UK due to immigration, new forms of cohabitation and increasing social mobility. Altschuler also considers the effects of HIV/AIDS on both family functioning and family configuration, illustrating it with research from the East African community in east London.

The book contains a number of chapters on methods of intervention and Jennie Lester focuses on the value of structured life review with the terminally ill. Life review is a valuable and innovative therapy which allows people to tell their story, to feel empowered and to find expression for the powerful feelings engendered when anticipating their own death. Lester has pioneered this technique in palliative care, and in Chapter 5 illustrates its use with powerful case histories and examples of her structured questionnaires.

In Chapter 6, Jan McLaren examines the effects of parental loss of a child aged between 1 and 25 years, within a western context. She explores similarities and differences experienced by parents, grandparents and siblings, identifying helpful interventions. The author, a person-centred counsellor and psychotherapist, uses her own perspective and the widening body of literature to bring a strong reflective analysis to this subject. Her work also draws upon her own qualitative research into the experience of bereaved parents as they tussle with what is described as the single worst experience of their lives. Making sense of the loss remains a central challenge to all such parents and families, along with finding an enduring place for the dead child within their lives (Klass 1997).

Grace H. Christ (Chapter 7) introduces interventions with bereaved children, based upon years of detailed and meticulous research in the USA. Her research and social work practice have enabled her to propose 'a two-dimensional model of childhood bereavement which incorporates both an ecological and developmental dimension'. Her work with children showing symptoms of traumatic stress following the 11 September 2001 attack on the New York World Trade Center led her to question the value of time-limited interventions and she proposes that both families and children may require multiple simultaneous interventions as well as the spread of support over time. Her chapter includes an excellent table of formally evaluated bereavement interventions, and she highlights the strengths and limitations of current research and suggests further research topics.

In Chapter 8, Peter Beresford, Suzy Croft, Lesley Adshead, Jean Walker and Karen Wilman highlight the contradictions within the field of palliative care in the UK concerning the involvement of service users. The authors differentiate between 'offering a voice' and 'accessing people's *own* voice' and emphasize the difference between a medical and a social model of palliative care. The further burdening of ill and vulnerable people is sometimes cited as a deterrent to active research, which is questioned by the authors, who stress the reciprocal nature of participation by service users at both a local and a strategic level.

In the UK there has been a movement, both social and political, towards the examination of social inclusion and exclusion. The terminally ill and bereaved experience multiple losses which are often coupled with increasing social isolation. Felicity Hearn examines this in Chapter 9 and provides us with a useful table that identifies social groups vulnerable to social exclusion. She challenges us to consider the issues by using practice examples that draw attention to some particularly vulnerable groups, for example, prisoners, the elderly in residential care, people with a learning disability, the mentally ill, and people who are excluded because of their ethnicity. Exclusion is further increased by poverty, which can be a major consequence of long periods of ill health and unemployment.

Several authors have discussed the effect of illness upon the whole family. In Chapter 10, Richard Harding focuses upon the needs of informal carers (usually family members). He uses research evidence to support the view that carers have unmet needs *and* they are often ambivalent about the care they provide. When their needs for support are assessed, few interventions are suggested. The research he quotes demonstrates that most people would prefer to die at home, but the number of cancer home deaths is less than 30 per cent. The reason for this discrepancy is neither medical- nor patient-related, but has more to do with social, physical, psychological, practical and emotional circumstances. There are some descriptive accounts of interventions for carers that Harding suggests lack rigorous evaluation. The author gives an account of a research study group intervention that he co-led. He concludes that there is little evidence that palliative care services provide effective support for informal carers.

Pam Firth's chapter (Chapter 11) on groupwork begins with a review of some well-known groupwork theories. She goes on to look at ideas from systemic theory and shows how they have influenced modern groupwork theorists within the UK and the USA. The practice examples demonstrate the enormous value of using groupwork as a method of intervention for adults and children who have been left disadvantaged and disempowered. Her emphasis on training, good leadership and supervision argues the need for groupwork training for nurses and doctors. Firth provides a clear discussion about the main practicalities of how to use groups effectively in palliative care but cautions that research into specific types of groupwork interventions and their timing is woefully lacking.

There is, as yet, little information on cross-cultural perspectives of loss and bereavement. In Chapter 12, Shirley Firth, drawing on her important research on cultural perspectives, emphasizes that we cannot rely on western ideas of 'normal' or 'pathological' grief. She surveys the current literature and discusses the expression of feelings, mourning and the role of meaning in loss, relating it to world cultures. Bereavement training and support must address the needs of minority ethnic people within western society. For example, appropriate education of those offering a service requires much greater commitment than is currently given. Training has to take into account 'transcultural studies from ethnographic and psychological perspectives and be committed to racial and cultural awareness'.

In the final chapter, the editors identify some of the important strands which have been developed by the contributors to this book. Loss, change and bereavement is a cyclical process: loss is inextricably interwoven into our lives.

References

Field, D. (2000) What do we mean by 'psychosocial'? A discussion paper on the use of the concept within palliative care. London: National Council for Hospice and Specialist Palliative Care Services. Briefing Paper No. 4.

Klass, D. (1997) Parental bereavement, in D. Klass, P. Silverman and S. Nickman (eds) Continuing Bonds: New Understandings of Grief. Washington: Taylor & Francis.

Sheldon, F. (2003) Social impact of advanced metastatic cancer, in M. Lloyd-Williams (ed.) Psychosocial Issues in Palliative Care. Oxford: Oxford University Press.

1 | The context of loss, change and bereavement in palliative care

Ann Quinn

Palliative care – in Britain as throughout the world – has now become synonymous with specialist care for those who are dying, encompassing physical, psychological, social and spiritual aspects and extending beyond death, since the focus is on the family as well as the patient. Thus care in bereavement is part of the remit as well as care of the dying.

(Currer 2001: 2)

Within palliative care services, death is seen as an integral part of life. Life itself, from all its aspects, forms the context of bereavement, loss and change. For the purposes of this chapter, I shall concentrate on some limited aspects from the early 1990s onwards, and within the UK: changed understandings of grief; the provision of palliative care and bereavement support; health and social care organization and policy. Such divisions are inevitably artificial; aspects interact, and are not nested neatly and hierarchically. Nor are these interactions confined to their UK setting: the understanding of grief and the development of bereavement services in the UK has been influenced by international perspectives and developments, amidst a growing awareness of cultural diversity.

At the centre of any consideration of context is a bereaved individual, facing loss and change, possibly grief. Grief can be searingly painful, but palliative care emphasizes its normality. In the face of grief, people are usually resilient, supported by family and friends, by informal social networks rather than formal bereavement services.

Changed understandings of grief

Grief is not an inevitable consequence of bereavement, loss and change. The meaning of the loss or change to an individual is critical in determining the nature of any grief response (Parkes 1993; Wortman *et al.* 1993; Neimeyer 2001). Bereavement and loss are not discrete events: they emerge from and interact with other life experiences. Current understanding also emphasizes the heterogeneity of individual responses, and the importance of social and cultural contexts (Stroebe *et al.* 2001a; Thompson 2002).

For about half a century leading up to the 1990s, there was a dominant understanding of grief. Stage and task models were based on the concept of grief work, detailing the process of grief for a bereaved person that resulted in detachment from the deceased and moving on to form new relationships (Lindemann 1944; Parkes 1996). Such models were strongly influenced by attachment theory (Bowlby 1969), and were developed to describe the experience of people who were bereaved. They were also widely applied to those who had experienced non-death losses. Such applicability was seen as a particular advantage of Worden's (1991) influential task model. The absence of grief in the face of a major loss was perceived as pathological, as was delayed or chronic grief (Middleton *et al.* 1993). While individual variation was acknowledged, models that were initially developed as flexible descriptions of grief were being applied prescriptively.

By the early 1990s this consensus was being challenged, by practitioners, researchers and, importantly, by bereaved people themselves. Writing in 1996, Walter considered this no mere shift in emphasis: 'The study of bereavement is currently in a revolutionary phase; it is no longer possible to ignore findings that do not fit the dominant model' (1996a: 10).

Traditional understanding held that bereaved people move from high distress to a resolution of grief. To do otherwise, whether by never showing distress or by maintaining an ongoing relationship with the deceased, was seen as abnormal and probably pathological. In their influential 1993 *Handbook*, Stroebe and colleagues gathered a body of research findings which did not support such beliefs (Stroebe *et al.* 1993). Stroebe had previously reviewed what she termed 'the grief work hypothesis', raising questions about the evidence base for the notion of working through grief (Stroebe 1992). In the handbook, Kaminer and Lavie (1993) reported findings demonstrating the value of repressing memories for Holocaust survivors, when earlier such repression would have been viewed as pathological. Wortman *et al.* summarized their findings from an extensive research programme into adjustment to loss and bereavement:

A substantial percentage of people do not appear to experience intense distress following a major loss. Instead, by as early as 1 month following the loss, there is marked variability in response. Moreover,

initial reactions appear to be highly predictive of long-term adjustment.

(Wortman *et al.* 1993: 355)

While some aspects of their findings were contested, their work was
influential. It highlighted the need to re-examine widespread assumptions.

Bereaved people themselves were also challenging some of the long-held
beliefs about grief. Particularly strong critiques of the way resolution was
formulated as a return to the state prior to bereavement came from parents
bereaved by the death of a child (Silverman and Klass 1996). Their voices
were heard directly – for example via such mutual help organizations as
Compassionate Friends, formed in 1969 to support parents who had lost a
child – or indirectly, via practitioners' accounts (Hindmarch 1993). Parents
did not wish to detach from a relationship with their child, nor did they see
a return to their pre-bereavement status as either possible or desirable.
Greater attention to children's experience of grief revealed similar themes:
bereaved of a parent, a child's understanding of the meaning of that loss
develops through life. Children also retain a sense of the presence of their
deceased parent in their life, a phenomenon labelled 'continuing bonds' by
Klass and colleagues (1996).

New models of grief have developed alongside such challenges. Classic
understandings of grief had a focus 'weighted towards the individual –
leading to an emphasis on the need for one-to-one counselling' (Currer
2001: 101). More recent models consider interpersonal as well as intra-
personal issues (Stroebe and Schut 1995; Walter 1996b; Kissane and Bloch
2002). Stroebe and Schut (1995, 2001) developed a dual process model
(DPM), which identifies two dimensions of experiencing loss: loss orientation with a focus on the past, and restoration orientation with a focus on
the present and the future. The term 'oscillation' is used to describe the
process of moving between these two dimensions. Both orientations are
necessary for adjustment. Oscillation also describes the process of moving
between confronting and avoiding these dimensions of loss. This model was
welcomed by palliative care practitioners as offering a new approach, one
which matched with their observations in practice. Silverman (Chapter 2 of
this book) considers the dual process model in more detail. For my purposes
here, it is important that this is a model which acknowledges diversity both
in terms of individual differences in the pattern of oscillation, and in terms
of gender and culture. Stroebe and Schut's own research showed that
women tended to be oriented more to loss, men to restoration; they note
also research evidence to suggest that different cultures may deem a particular orientation more appropriate. This model also acknowledges the
practical tasks that need to be undertaken in coping with grief, in attending
to life changes and changing social roles and relationships as well as the
emotional grief work.

Walter's (1996b) biographical model has not been as widely influential as the dual process model. Nevertheless, his emphasis on the social context of grief rather than the intrapersonal emotions, and on the importance of the bereaved talking to others about the dead, resonated with many practitioners. But there was some discord. Bereavement counsellors, both within and outside palliative care, felt that they had been misrepresented in some of the challenges to the traditional models. Presenting a counsellor's perspective, McLaren was critical of Walter: 'he assumes that all (or most) bereavement counsellors uphold the conventional wisdom of bereavement theory' (1998: 276). She described her counselling practice as based on a person-centred approach (see Rogers 1951). This approach underpinned a counselling style which was not confined by prevailing bereavement theory but acknowledged bereaved people as the experts, capable of finding their own answers. Many offering bereavement support within palliative care would echo her account of a greater diversity in practice than critiques of bereavement counselling acknowledge (Parkes *et al.* 1996).

Change has been less explored within palliative care than either bereavement or loss. Marris's early work seeing loss in relation to change was influential (Marris 1986), particularly through Parkes' conceptualization of psychosocial transitions (Parkes 1993). The emphasis on the meaning of loss or change, its impact on the individual's assumptive world, helped provide a structure for translating an understanding of grief derived from bereavement to a wider range of non-death-related loss and change. Silverman (1988, 2000) saw change as an integral part of the grief process, and her research did much to place grief in a context of changing social relationships and roles. Neimeyer's work on meaning reconstruction places change as a central feature of grieving: 'this often effortful attempt to reconfigure a viable self and world in light of the loss proceeds on deeply personal and intricately social levels simultaneously' (Neimeyer and Anderson 2002: 47).

'Our descriptions of grief have far outstripped our ability to explain it' (Stroebe *et al.* 2001b: 746). What we do know leads to caution in extrapolating understandings from bereavement research – from death-related loss and change – into the wider ranges of non-death loss and change. We need to tease out the similarities and differences between (and within) bereavement, loss and change (Harvey 1998).

Most palliative care practitioners welcomed the new perspectives: although some argued that they had always endorsed the tenets of the 'revolution'. The emphasis on diversity chimed with their concern to extend bereavement services to those groups at risk of marginalization: people with learning disabilities, mental health problems or dementia; homosexual or extramarital partners; people from other cultures. Rosenblatt, who has written widely about cross-cultural variations in grief, conveyed the sense of a world that may well be startlingly different from our preconceptions, and concluded: 'It pays to treat everyone as though he or she were from a different culture. The cross-cultural emphasis, in fact, is a kind of metaphor. To help effectively, we must overcome our presuppositions and struggle to understand people on their own terms' (Rosenblatt 1993: 18). This belief in the importance of meeting people on their own terms is highly congruent with values held within palliative care. What is perhaps less well recognized is the personal struggle it can entail. Gunaratnam has drawn on her hospice-based research to describe the emotional labour inherent in working with difference, the practitioner's subjective experience of anti-oppressive practice (Gunaratnam *et al.* 1998; Gunaratnam 2002). She also emphasized that acknowledgment of diversity should not overshadow an awareness of socially patterned inequality. Desai and Bevan (2002: 60) note that

> it is only relatively recently that it has been recognized that there is a need for an anti-racist (rather than simply ethnically-sensitive) approach to be established in order to do justice to the complexities of the experience of loss on the part of people who have to contend with the pressures of racism in addition to the pain of their particular loss or losses.

The social structuring of disadvantage and exclusion was neglected in traditional approaches to loss and grief; Hearn (Chapter 9 of this book) explores current practice which pays due attention to the needs of people at risk of exclusion.

The new understandings of grief were disseminated among palliative care practitioners through the Bereavement Research Forum, developed early in the 1990s; through the biennial congresses of the European Association of Palliative Care which started in 1990; and via meetings of their various professional associations. Palliative care practitioners in turn offered education and training on bereavement and loss to other health and social care professionals, contributed to the research base and published in this area. Such activity both reflected and contributed to the acceptance of providing family and bereavement support as an integral part of palliative care.

The provision of palliative care and bereavement support

Specialist palliative care services

Bereavement support within palliative care can be seen as starting before death, at the point of referral to the palliative care service when the needs of family and friends are assessed. In the UK, bereavement support after the death is delivered both by professionals as a continuation of their care to patients and families – 'follow-up' bereavement support – and by teams set up specifically to provide a bereavement service. Such teams are frequently staffed by volunteers trained and supervised by professionals. The inter-action between a palliative care service and the bereavement service within it is fluid. There is evidence that good palliative care of dying people has an impact on the distress experienced later by their bereaved survivors (Grande et al. 2000; Kissane and Bloch 2002). Palliative care can thus be seen as part of bereavement care.

As of January 2004, there were 217 palliative care units, and 30 children's hospices in the UK; 64 of these were NHS units and the rest voluntary services. There were 356 home care teams, plus 94 Hospice at Home teams; 258 day care units; 72 hospital support nurses and 281 hospital support teams (Brasch 2004). Two national cancer charities – Macmillan Cancer Relief and Marie Curie Cancer Care – have played a major role in the development of these services, often in partnership with the public sector. In her characteristically informative overview of the development of palliative care, Sheldon (1997) also emphasized the part played by local voluntary effort. She concluded: 'The rapid and opportunistic development of palliative care services complementary to the existing primary and secondary health care services produced considerable differences in organisation and remit between palliative care services' (1997: 40).

There are similarly wide differences in the organization and remit of bereavement services within palliative care, but in some ways we know little about the nature of bereavement support. This may seem surprising in the light of accounts in later chapters of this book and elsewhere, with practitioners discussing their work in detail. What we do not know is how representative such services are.

Hospice Information produces an annual directory of all hospice and palliative care services in the UK and Ireland. Each entry notes whether or not a bereavement service is offered, but the nature of this bereavement service is not identified. Payne and Relf (1994) undertook a postal survey of the 397 palliative care services and teams identified in the 1992 directory. They aimed to determine the nature and extent of services provided for bereaved adults and to investigate how units assessed the need for bereavement follow-up. A total of 187 questionnaires were returned, a response rate of 47 per cent. Of those, 84 per cent were providing bereavement follow-up, and a further 7 per cent planned some form of bereavement service. Their study reinforced the belief that there is no clear rationale for the delivery of bereavement services: only 25 per cent of the units that responded undertook formal risk assessment procedures. Most services relied on clinical experience rather than standardized measures to target support. The authors commented: 'Experience and instinct should not be denigrated. Parkes found that nurses' intuitive feelings were the best predictors of outcome. However, reliance on experience raises a number of issues. How do we ensure criteria are being used consistently? How can experience be passed on?' (Payne and Relf 1994: 297).

A current research project is investigating the bereavement support being provided to adults by hospices and specialist palliative care services (Payne et al. 2004). Of the 301 UK palliative care units and teams listed in the 2002 directory as providing bereavement services to adults, 249 (83 per cent) replied to a survey questionnaire. Preliminary findings were that the most common type of service was individual support; 68 per cent of bereavement services involved volunteers; there was considerable variation within services as to the numbers of service users, length of service, and whether or not there was any needs assessment; the 'primary qualification' of those offering bereavement support was nursing in 36 per cent of services, social work in 21 per cent, and counselling in 18.5 per cent. Surprising, but also of concern, was the finding that of those services which did use volunteers, 5 per cent did not offer them any support and a significant minority of services (13 per cent) did not offer supervision to paid workers. We need more such studies, to build a comprehensive picture of the services available.

Services offered to bereaved people are highly variable and include individual visits, group sessions and telephone contact; cards may be sent on the anniversary of the death and memorial services held to commemorate those who have died during a particular period (Sheldon 1997). Most units provide written information in a leaflet, explaining common responses to bereavement, how bereaved people can obtain help from their service, and listing local and national sources of support. Such information encourages people to self-refer if they feel in need of bereavement help. Services may also operate on an outreach basis, contacting those assessed as at risk of a poor bereavement outcome or those groups who might not otherwise find the service accessible, such as children or people with learning disabilities.

The definition of many terms used is unclear: bereavement services may provide bereavement support or bereavement counselling, offered either by a professional using counselling skills or someone called variously a bereavement counsellor, a bereavement befriender or a bereavement supporter. Services may have a psychotherapeutic focus, but in many cases they are offering a mix of practical assistance and social support as well as using counselling skills (Parkes et al. 1996). This distinction between being a counsellor and using counselling skills is clear conceptually, but not necessarily in practice. A related distinction used to be made between grief therapy, helping people with abnormal or complicated grief reactions, and grief counselling which helps facilitate normal grief (Worden 1991). This distinction is not currently made within palliative care, reflecting widespread reservations about the concept of abnormal grief (Middleton et al. 1993).

Payne and Relf (1994) noted that risk assessment tools were unsatisfactory;

this remains true. As well as methodological weaknesses (W. Stroebe and Schut 2001) there are conceptual difficulties. When used in practice, it can be unclear whether the risk being assessed – poor bereavement outcome – refers to the grief process itself or to health outcomes. Similarly, the evaluation of bereavement interventions is methodologically complex: 'A substantial number of grief intervention efficacy studies have resulted in disappointing, sometimes even negative results' (Schut *et al.* 2001: 705). Under a heading of 'When (not) to Intervene', Stroebe *et al.* (2001b: 761) summarize the current consensus that 'counselling and therapy are only needed for a minority of high-risk bereaved people'. They cite Parkes in support:

> There is no evidence that all bereaved people will benefit from counselling and research has shown no benefits to arise from the routine referral of people to counselling for no other reason than that they have suffered a bereavement. Such routine offers of help may cause family members and others to feel superfluous, and to back off when they are most needed.
>
> (Parkes 1998: 18)

Unfortunately, we do not have the ability to distinguish that minority of high-risk bereaved people reliably.

Other bereavement services

Considerable differences in organization and remit are evident in other bereavement services in the community: Faulkner (1993: 73) refers to a 'hotch potch' of services. There is, however, some coordination. Organizations involved in bereavement care nationally, including the National Council for Hospices and Specialist Palliative Care Services, are cooperating on a project to develop bereavement standards. It is intended to include core standards translated into 'delivery contexts' such as befriending, counselling, facilitated groups and telephone support (Bereavement Care Standards 2001). The aim is to produce agreed definitions of terms such as 'support', 'befriending' and 'counselling'. Success in this will greatly assist in identifying the nature of current bereavement services.

A voluntary organization, the National Association of Bereavement Services used to provide a directory of all bereavement services; it has, however, closed because of lack of funding. Without a directory of bereavement services more generally, it is hard to know their numbers nationally, or their geographical spread. We know that the largest national bereavement charity – Cruse Bereavement Care – has 178 branches throughout the UK, and that the London Bereavement Network, for example, lists 25 services within London boroughs. Other cities and regions also have bereavement networks offering some local listings and coordination. There is more coordination of bereavement support services for children. The Childhood Bereavement Network was established in 2001 as a membership organization for services providing bereavement support to children and young people; it currently has 127 members. Rolls (2004) is undertaking a study to explore UK childhood bereavement services, examining the type of service organization, the nature and focus of service provision, and describing children's and families' experiences of using such services. Complementing Payne and colleagues' study of specialist palliative care bereavement services for adults, Rolls's study will significantly extend our knowledge of the nature of bereavement support in the UK.

The standards project estimates that 80 per cent of bereavement support is delivered by the voluntary sector, and 90 per cent by volunteers (Bereavement Care Standards 2001). New services are constantly developing: there is growing use of website chatrooms and message boards by bereaved people, and bereavement services are beginning to offer email advice via their websites. Mutual or self-help groups are widely used by bereaved people (Lieberman, 1993). Hockey and Small (2001) note how one such organization, Cruse Bereavement Care, has changed over the years. Originally, Cruse provided mutual help to widows facing the myriad practical tasks and changes following bereavement; now it provides counselling, with a focus on individual emotions. Hockey and Small link this shift to Walter's (1999) analysis of the way bereavement services 'police' or regulate grief. Without a clearer picture of the nature of bereavement services, the justice of such criticism cannot be properly evaluated.

The numerous public sector workers offering assistance at the time of death are often ignored when considering bereavement services. There are bereavement officers based in local authority cemeteries and within NHS hospitals. Their role is usually predominantly administrative, providing information, helping people with the necessary practical tasks following a death, and directing bereaved people towards sources of help. As with other bereavement services, the backgrounds of the people providing the service are very variable, as is the nature of any training or support received.

Health and social care

The structure and organization of health and social care in the UK has been subject to much change over the past decade. Public sector reform is a political priority. Reorganizations, policy statements, guidelines and regulations have proliferated: 'Policy flowing from central government is generating a new terminology, changing responsibilities and introducing innovatory practice' (Bytheway *et al.* 2002: xi). It has also generated weariness in the face of what is seen as constant change, and the criticism that politicians are meddling in health care services on a day-to-day basis (Dewar 2003). A similar policy avalanche confronts social care: Douglas and Philpott (1998) note that over a hundred new volumes of guidance on social care were issued by the government between 1990 and 1995.

Health and social care are structured separately in the UK (except for in Northern Ireland). Local authorities are responsible for statutory social services in their area, funded predominantly by a grant from central government. These statutory services are supplemented by voluntary and private agencies. As Currer (2001) notes, this separation of health and social care can have important consequences. Many dying or bereaved people require services from both sectors. The need for integration is widely acknowledged, and the government has called for more collaboration and joint working (Department of Health 1998). Lewis is sceptical: 'Health and local authorities have always battled over their responsibilities and the battles have been fuelled by the financial implications of admitting responsibility and by professional ideas as to what health and social care are all about' (2002: 313). 'Continuing care', the long-term care of chronically ill or slowly dying people, is one such battleground. The decision as to which sector is responsible has profound financial implications for service users: health care is free at the point of use, social care provision is charged on the basis of a means-test of users.

For much of the UK, but not Northern Ireland, palliative care services are organized within cancer networks. These recently developed structures bring together health service commissioners and providers, the voluntary sector and local authorities in a particular area: typically a network serves a population of between 1 million and 2 million people (Department of Health 2003). There are 34 networks in England, 3 in Wales and 3 in Scotland. The strategic planning of bereavement support should take place within the cancer networks. Health and social care services within Northern Ireland continue to be organized within four Health and Social Services Boards; Northern Ireland integrated health and the personal social services some time ago. Strategic Health Authorities (England), regional offices (Wales) and NHS Boards (Scotland) manage local health services, integrating primary care services with secondary and more specialist services. Devolution has had an impact, with the four regions of the UK developing increasingly divergent structures and policies.

Despite continuous organizational change and policy innovation, some aspects of palliative care and bereavement services remain relevant: the extension of palliative care to all dying or bereaved people; the funding of palliative care and bereavement services; evidence-based practice; and user involvement.

Extending palliative care

Specialist palliative care services are disproportionately available to those with a diagnosis of cancer, but even within this group only a small number receive palliative care and there is inequitable access to services. The NHS Cancer Plan (Department of Health 2000) pledged additional money to increase equity of access, and further money is being made available to train district nurses and other community staff in palliative care.

Guidelines have been produced to improve supportive and palliative care for adults with cancer (NICE 2004). The reference to supportive care draws on the concept of a spectrum of palliative care provision. The National Council for Hospice and Specialist Palliative Care Services (NCHSPCS) employs 'supportive care' as an umbrella term for all services, generalist and specialist, that may be required to support people with cancer and their carers from the time that cancer is suspected. Supportive care is the responsibility of all health and social care professionals, rather than a distinct speciality (NCHSPCS 2002). The NICE guidelines include bereavement care as an integral part of the services needed by families and carers of a person with cancer.

The moral case for extending palliative care beyond cancer is clear (George and Sykes 1997). The UK Department of Health has recognized that palliative care should be available on the basis of need, not diagnosis; this is underlined by the recognition within National Service Frameworks of the palliative care needs of elderly people and those with coronary heart disease (NCHSPCS 1998, 2001). As Clayson argues, however, the new funding for palliative care is tied to cancer money, and is not for expanding services to include non-cancer illnesses: 'There is an urgent need for an interim agreement to establish the way forward for funding all end-of-life care' (2003: 14).

The funding of palliative care and bereavement services

Sheldon (1997) noted how the mixed economy of care could make it difficult to identify how palliative care services are funded. Department of Health figures claim that, on average, 28 per cent of the running costs of adult hospices are covered by state funding, and 5 per cent of the costs of children's hospices (Clayson 2003). More funding for specialist palliative care services was signalled in the NHS Cancer Plan (Department of Health 2000). Clayson, a trustee of Help the Hospices, expresses some concern: 'The new money has strings attached. ... The challenge is to ensure the new funding agreements allow hospices to develop while preserving the principles of hospice care and without compromising their independence, flexibility and sensitivity to local needs' (Clayson 2003: 14). Her concerns echo the earlier views of Biswas (1993), who feared that government funding could distort care, resulting in 'medicalization' of dying.

Specialist palliative care services usually have a more stable financial situation than many of the other bereavement services. London Bereavement Network (LBN) highlights the issues: 'A "typical" bereavement service which belongs to LBN may receive a third of its funding from the local borough and a third from the health authority, both cut by at least 10% from the year before; and a lot of time and energy has to be spent gathering together the remaining third of funds needed' (London Bereavement Network 2001). Continuity of funding is difficult to achieve. This reflects a broader problem for voluntary sector agencies whereby funding bodies will support new initiatives for a fixed term, but not provide the funding necessary for agencies to continue their core functions (Quinn et al. 2003).

Evidence-based practice

The need to subject assumptions about the nature of grief to empirical verification was discussed earlier. This partly reflects a government-sponsored movement towards evidence-based practice in health and social care. NICE – the National Institute for Clinical Excellence – was set up in 1999 as part of the NHS; its role is to provide patients, health professionals and the public with 'authoritative, robust and reliable guidance' on current best practice (NICE 2003).

The Social Care Institute for Excellence (SCIE) was established in 2001, with the task of gathering and publicizing knowledge about how to make social care services better (SCIE).

It is clearly desirable to base practice on evidence. Criticism centres on what evidence 'counts', and the primacy given to randomized controlled trials. There is a danger of relying on readily quantifiable outcomes of intervention, and basing performance indicators on such measures. We need to develop research methods that are congruent with exploring people's experience of bereavement, loss and change, and which can more effectively evaluate the complex interventions involved in palliative care. Machin (Chapter 3 of this book) explores this in more detail.

User involvement

Another government-sponsored movement, user involvement in services (Department of Health 2001) has the ability to counteract a trend towards 'medicalization' resulting from the standardization of services which could stem from the pressures of evidence-based practice. Users involved in research, for example, have emphasized the importance of process, the nature of the relationship between staff and service users: 'no good outcomes without good process' (Fisher 2002). Users' perspectives on evaluation challenge the reliance on standardized outcomes.

In considering user involvement and partnership, it is important to distinguish between management- or service-centred approaches and truly participative user-centred involvement where service users' objectives and priorities become the organization's objectives and priorities (Robson *et al.* 2003). A user-centred approach puts patient and carer at the heart of services, congruent with the values of palliative care.

Conclusion

If there is one theme underlying these different aspects of the context of loss, change and bereavement in palliative care, it is diversity: diversity in the grief response of those who face bereavement, loss and change; diversity in the bereavement services available; diversity in the organization and policies of health and social care.

A bereaved person experiencing grief is at the centre of any understanding of context. This person may also be a member of social networks which include other people facing grief. Bereavement services within palliative care aim to respond to the needs of such diverse individuals and communities. There is a growing recognition of the complex social structures and power relations which affect the experience of bereavement.

Bereavement services require financial resources, but current funding frameworks are fragmented and inadequate. The policy context of performance targets and league tables is a potential threat to the more holistic culture of palliative care, but the impetus towards user involvement is a welcome opportunity. The people we are trying to help are the most important source of our understanding and for shaping service priorities: 'Our active curiosity and genuine interest are of the utmost importance' (Rosenblatt 1993: 17).

Palliative care services aim not only to disseminate good practice within their specialist sector but also to influence the mainstream health and social care settings in which the majority of people experience bereavement. This book is part of that process.

References

Bereavement Care Standards (2001) UK project *Standards for Bereavement Care in the UK*. Available at www.bereavement.org.uk/standards/index.asp (accessed December 2003).

Biswas, B. (1993) The medicalisation of dying: a nurse's view, in D. Clark (ed.) *The Future for Palliative Care*. Buckingham: Open University Press.

Bowlby, J. (1969) *Attachment and Loss. Vol. 1: Attachment*. London: Basic Books.

Brasch, S. (ed.) (2004) *Hospice Directory 2004. Hospices and Palliative Care Services in the United Kingdom and Ireland*. London: Hospice Information.

Bytheway, B., Bacigalupo, V., Bornat, J., Johnson, J. and Spurr, S. (eds) (2002) Preface, in *Understanding Care, Welfare and Community: A Reader*. London: Routledge.

Clayson, H. (2003) Hospices to fortune, *BMA news*, 22 February, pp. 13–14.

Currer, C. (2001) *Responding to Grief: Dying, Bereavement and Social Care*. Basingstoke: Palgrave.

Department of Health (1998) *Modernising Social Services*, Cm. 4169. London: HMSO.

Department of Health (2000) *The NHS Cancer Plan: A Plan for Investment, A Plan for Reform*. London: Department of Health.

Department of Health (2001) *New Arrangements for Patient and Public Involvement*. London: Department of Health.

Department of Health (2003) *The NHS Cancer Plan Three Year Progress Report: Maintaining the Momentum*. London: Department of Health.

Desai, S. and Bevan, D. (2002) Race and culture, in N. Thompson (ed.) *Loss and Grief: A Guide for Human Service Practitioners*. Basingstoke: Palgrave.

Dewar, S. (2003) *Government and the NHS – Time for a New Relationship?* London: The King's Fund.

Douglas, A. and Philpot, T. (1998) *Caring and Coping: A Guide to Social Services*. London: Routledge.

Faulkner, A. (1993) Developments in bereavement services, in D. Clark (ed.) *The Future for Palliative Care: Issues of Policy and Practice*. Buckingham: Open University Press.

Fisher, M. (2002) The role of service users in problem formulation and technical aspects of social research, *Social Work Education*, 21(3): 305–12.

George, R. and Sykes, J. (1997) Beyond cancer?, in D. Clark, J. Hockley and S. Ahmedzai (eds) *New Themes in Palliative Care*. Buckingham: Open University Press.

Grande, G., Todd, C.J., Barclay, S.I.G. and Farquhar, M.C. (2000) A randomised controlled trial of a hospital at home service for the terminally ill, *Palliative Medicine*, 14: 375–85.

Gunaratnam, Y. (2002) Whiteness and emotions in social care, in B. Bytheway, V. Bacigalupo, J. Bornat, J. Johnson and S. Spurr (eds) *Understanding Care, Welfare and Community: A Reader*. London: Routledge.

Gunaratnam, Y., Bremner, I., Pollock, L. and Weir, C. (1998) Anti-discrimination, emotions and professional practice, *European Journal of Palliative Care*, 5(4): 122–4.

Harvey, J.H. (ed.) (1998) *Perspectives on Loss: A Sourcebook*. Philadelphia: Brunner Routledge

Hindmarch, C. (1993) *Death of a Child*. Oxford: Radcliffe Medical Press.

Hockey, J. and Small, N. (2001) Discourse into practice: the production of bereavement care, in J. Hockey, J. Katz and N. Small (eds) *Grief, Mourning and Death Ritual*. Buckingham: Open University Press.

Kaminer, H. and Lavie, P. (1993) Sleep and dreams in well-adjusted and less adjusted Holocaust survivors, in M. Stroebe, W. Stroebe and R. Hansson (eds)

Handbook of Bereavement: Theory, Research and Intervention. Cambridge: Cambridge University Press.

Kissane, D. and Bloch, S. (2002) *Family Focused Grief Therapy*. Buckingham: Open University Press

Klass, D., Silverman, P. and Nickman, S. (eds) (1996) *Continuing Bonds: New Understandings of Grief*. Washington, DC: Taylor & Francis.

Lewis, J. (2002) The boundary between health and social care for older people, in B. Bytheway, V. Bacigalupo, J. Bornat, J. Johnson and S. Spurr (eds) *Understanding Care, Welfare and Community: A Reader*. London: Routledge.

Lieberman, M.A. (1993) Bereavement self-help groups, in M. Stroebe, W. Stroebe and R. Hansson (eds) *Handbook of Bereavement: Theory, Research and Intervention*. Cambridge: Cambridge University Press.

Lindemann, E. (1944) Symptomatology and management of acute grief, *American Journal of Psychiatry*, 101: 141–8.

London Bereavement Network (2001) *What do we do?* Available at www. bereavement.org.uk/about/whatdowedo.asp (accessed December 2003).

McLaren, J. (1998) A new understanding of grief: a counsellor's perspective, *Mortality*, 3(3): 275–90.

Marris, P. (1986) *Loss and Change*, rev. edn. London: Routledge.

Middleton, W., Raphael, B., Martinek, N. and Misso, V. (1993) Pathological grief reactions, in M. Stroebe, W. Stroebe and R. Hansson (eds) *Handbook of Bereavement: Theory, Research and Intervention*. Cambridge: Cambridge University Press.

NCHSPCS (1998) *Reaching Out: Specialist Palliative Care for Adults with Non-malignant Diseases*. London: National Council for Hospice and Specialist Palliative Care Services.

NCHSPCS (2001) *Building on Success: Strategic Agenda 2001–2004*. Available at www.hospice.spc.council.org.uk/publications/otherdocs.htm (accessed December 2003).

NCHSPCS (2002) *Definitions of Supportive and Palliative Care: A Discussion Paper*. London: National Council for Hospice and Specialist Palliative Care Services.

Neimeyer, R.A. (ed.) (2001) *Meaning Reconstruction and the Experience of Loss*. Washington, DC: American Psychological Association.

Neimeyer, R.A. and Anderson, A. (2002) Meaning reconstruction theory, in N. Thompson (ed.) *Loss and Grief: A Guide for Human Services Practitioners*. Basingstoke: Palgrave.

NICE (2004) *Improving Supportive and Palliative Care for Adults with Cancer*. Available at http://www.nice.org.uk/cat.asp?c=110005 (accessed March 2004).

NICE (2003) *About NICE*. Available at www.nice.org.uk/cat.asp?c=137 (accessed December 2003).

Parkes, C.M. (1993) Bereavement as a psychosocial transition: processes of adaptation to change, in M. Stroebe, W. Stroebe and R. Hansson (eds) *Handbook of Bereavement: Theory, Research and Intervention*. Cambridge: Cambridge University Press.

Parkes, C.M. (1996) *Bereavement: Studies of Grief in Adult Life*, 3rd edn. London: Routledge.

Parkes, C.M. (1998) Editorial, *Bereavement Care*, 17: 18.

Parkes, C.M., Relf, M. and Couldrick, A. (1996) *Counselling in Terminal Care and Bereavement*. Leicester: British Psychological Society.

Payne, S. and Relf, M. (1994) The assessment of need for bereavement follow-up in palliative and hospice care, *Palliative Medicine*, 8: 291–7.

Payne, S., Field, D., Relf, M. and Reid, D. (2004) Hospice-based bereavement services: preliminary results of a UK postal survey. Oral presentation, 5th Palliative Care Congress, University of Warwick, UK, 18 March, *Palliative Medicine*, 18(2): 151–2.

Quinn, A., Snowling, A. and Denicolo, P. (2003) *Older People's Perspectives: Devising Information, Advice and Advocacy Services*. York: Joseph Rowntree Foundation.

Robson, P., Begum, N. and Lock, M. (2003) *Developing User Involvement: Working towards User-centred Practice in Voluntary Organisations*. York: Joseph Rowntree Foundation.

Rogers, C.R. (1951) *Client-centred Therapy*. Boston, MA: Houghton-Mifflin.

Rolls, L. (2004) UK childhood bereavement services. Workshop at the 5th Palliative Care Congress, University of Warwick, UK, 19 March.

Rosenblatt, P. (1993) Cross-cultural variation in the experience, expression, and understanding of grief, in D.P. Irish, K.F. Lundquist and V.J. Nelson (eds) *Ethnic Variations in Dying, Death and Grief: Diversity in Universality*. Washington, DC: Taylor & Francis.

Schut, H., Stroebe, M.S., Van den Bout, J. and Terheggen, M. (2001) The efficacy of bereavement interventions: determining who benefits, in M. Stroebe, R. Hansson, W. Stroebe and H. Schut (eds) *Handbook of Bereavement Research: Consequences, Coping and Care*. Washington, DC: American Psychological Association.

SCIE (n.d.) *SCIE's Work*. Available at http://www.scie.org.uk/scieswork/scieswork.htm (accessed December 2003).

Sheldon, F. (1997) *Psychosocial Palliative Care: Good Practice in the Care of the Dying and Bereaved*. Cheltenham: Stanley Thornes.

Silverman, P.R. (1988) In search of new selves: accommodating to widowhood, in L.A. Bond and B. Wagner (eds) *Families in Transition: Primary Programs that Work*. Newbury Park, CA: Sage.

Silverman, P.R. (2000) *Never Too Young to Know: Death in Children's Lives*. New York: Oxford University Press.

Silverman, P.R. and Klass, D. (1996) Introduction: What's the problem? in D. Klass, P. Silverman and S. Nickman (eds) *Continuing Bonds: New Understandings of Grief*. Washington, DC: Taylor & Francis.

Stroebe, M. (1992) Coping with bereavement: a review of the grief work hypothesis, *Omega*, 26(1): 19–42.

Stroebe, M. and Schut, H. (1995) The dual process model of coping with loss. Paper presented at the International Work Group on Death, Dying and Bereavement, St Catherine's College, Oxford, 26–29 June.

Stroebe, M. and Schut, H. (2001) Models of coping with bereavement: a review, in M. Stroebe, R. Hansson, W. Stroebe and H. Schut (eds) *Handbook of Bereavement Research: Consequences, Coping and Care*. Washington, DC: American Psychological Association.

Stroebe, M., Stroebe, W. and Hansson, R. (eds) (1993) *Handbook of Bereavement:*

Theory, Research and Intervention. Cambridge: Cambridge University Press.

Stroebe, M., Hansson, R., Stroebe, W. and Schut, H. (2001a) Introduction: concepts and issues in contemporary research in bereavement, in M. Stroebe, R. Hansson, W. Stroebe and H. Schut (eds) *Handbook of Bereavement Research: Consequences, Coping and Care.* Washington, DC: American Psychological Association.

Stroebe, M., Hansson, R., Stroebe, W. and Schut, H. (2001b) Future directions for bereavement research, in M. Stroebe, R. Hansson, W. Stroebe and H. Schut (eds) *Handbook of Bereavement Research: Consequences, Coping and Care.* Washington, DC: American Psychological Association.

Stroebe, W. and Schut, H. (2001) Risk factors in bereavement outcome: a methodological and empirical review, in M. Stroebe, R. Hansson, W. Stroebe and H. Schut (eds) *Handbook of Bereavement Research: Consequences, Coping and Care.* Washington, DC: American Psychological Association.

Thompson, N. (ed.) (2002) Introduction, in *Loss and grief: A Guide for Human Services Practitioners.* Basingstoke: Palgrave.

Walter, T. (1996a) Bereavement models, *Progress in Palliative Care*, 4(1): 9–11.

Walter, T. (1996b) A new model of grief: bereavement and biography. *Mortality*, 1(1): 7–25.

Walter, T. (1999) *On Bereavement: The Culture of Grief.* Buckingham: Open University Press.

Worden, J.W. (1991) *Grief Counselling and Grief Therapy: A Handbook for the Mental Health Practitioner*, 2nd edn. London: Routledge.

Wortman, C.B., Silver, R.C. and Kessler, R.C. (1993) Adjustment to bereavement, in M. Stroebe, W. Stroebe and R. Hansson (eds) *Handbook of Bereavement: Theory, Research and Intervention.* Cambridge: Cambridge University Press.

2 Mourning: a changing view

Phyllis R. Silverman

This chapter uses a social constructivist perspective to provide an overview of how grief has been viewed in western society over the past century. Theories of grief have evolved leading to the observation that grief is not an illness from which people can recover. A key assumption of the chapter is that lived human experiences cannot be fixed. People are changed and they adapt to a new situation introduced by the death. The chapter begins by presenting a socially constructed view of grief. Using this lens, the decline of ritual during the twentieth century is discussed and various theories that have developed are described, building on Bowlby's (1980) concepts of attachment that bring in to the discourse a relational view of grief that involves continuing relationships with the deceased as well. Concepts of stress and coping are introduced to look at adaptive strategies mourners use.

A socially constructed view of grief

As we think about how people react to death, we recognize how varied these reactions have been over time and in various settings. We are looking at socially shaped ideas and assumptions subject to historical and cultural changes (Charmaz 1994; Stroebe *et al.* 1996; Walter 1999; Rosenblatt 2001). This concept of social construction suggests that mourning behaviours, while evolving from what has happened in earlier periods, reflect the values and attitudes of the time, place and context in which they are occurring. Rosenblatt (2001) observed that in a socially constructed view of the world everything can be seen as relative, so that it is difficult to define universal aspects of human behaviour. However, the fact that everyone dies is not socially constructed; we all have this in common. Neither is the fact that people react to death, socially constructed. This is a constant in every human society (Fulton 1965). However, *how* we react, that is, how we give meaning and direction to these events, is socially constructed. Every society and faith system has developed some way of integrating the reality of death into its belief system and way of life. It is these systems and beliefs that have changed considerably over the centuries. Thus, the attitudes and values of the society we live in provide direction for how we understand illness and health, how we define our purpose and place in the world, and how death and grief fit into this picture. These attitudes and values affect how we relate not only to ourselves but also to others, and how we give these experiences meaning. These ways of making meaning cannot be seen as isolated personal variables without reference to the historical, social and economic context of the time. A community's grief is invariably framed in a language compatible with the belief system of that society.

An example of this community process is documented by van Gennep (1960), an anthropologist writing in the early part of the twentieth century. He described mourning traditions in the communities he studied. He identified a multi-stage process of mourning, clearly stated in the communities' tradition, marking a rite of passage separating the living and the dead. Van Gennep observed that, in these communities, the initial focus was on the burial of the dead; mourners then visualize the dead person at rest in the land of the deceased from which there is no return, and finally there is a severing of ties with the deceased – a cessation of the role obligations that kept alive the deceased's involvement with the living. In many societies the rituals of mourning differentiate the duties of the mourner from those who are not mourning. For the mourners (and there is rarely a single mourner), daily routines are interrupted and behaviour changes are legitimated. In time, there are rituals of re-entry or reintegration into the community. Participating in these rituals shows solidarity with the social group of which the mourner is a part. Rosenblatt *et al.* (1976), in an anthropological review of bereavement practices in several less developed communities, identified a designated 'ritual specialist' whose task it is to guide the mourner through their mourning to a different place in society.

Decline of ritual

Another way of studying the rituals and beliefs associated with death and bereavement is to ask: what voices influence this culture and what do they have to say? There has been a dramatic change over the past 100 years in whose voices are heard. Explaining human behaviour around death and bereavement is no longer the prerogative of philosophers and clergymen and certain other members of the community. Gorer (1965) pointed to how mourning traditions had disappeared. He observed that, until the twentieth century, religious faith and ritual played an important part in helping people give expression and direction to their grief, including ways to mediate between the living and the dead. Gorer noted that the focus for mourners was on restraint, making the pain and sadness associated with loss a personal and private matter.

Over the twentieth century we moved from a time when communal rituals and practices, and religious beliefs, framed the mourners' behaviour to a time when the focus was (and still is) almost solely on the individual, their inner feelings and personal reactions. In western society, in the twentieth century, both the physical and the social sciences have had an important impact on religious philosophy that resulted in limiting its influence on where it fits into people's lives. Belief in an afterlife was pushed to the background and the value of ritual was minimized (Parsons 1994), so that neither played an active role in consoling or guiding the behaviour of the bereaved.

Psychological view of human behaviour

For the most part, contemporary views of grief have been framed by modern psychological theories and it is the voice of the psychologists and health care professionals that we hear. During the twentieth century we have witnessed what Meyer (1988) called the creation of the modern psychological individual. Meyer sees the qualities that define this individual as related to the complex social changes taking place in the western economic, cultural and political systems that foster the ideology of individualism with an emphasis on a scientific approach to understanding human behaviour. Psychological theories focus on the individual's responsibility for his/her own inner psyche, as well as that of his/her children. When the needs of the bereaved are framed in psychological terms, we focus primarily on the inner life of an individual, and this inner life is where researchers and clinicians have looked to understand any given person's reactions to a death. Coincidently, individual responses are framed in the language of illness so that mourners look for a way of recovering from this condition. In the twentieth century, death has been viewed as a medical failure and this has also framed our understanding of grief. Like death, grieving was separated from the normal life cycle and became something to avoid. By the middle of the twentieth century, mourning had become sanitized. As a consequence, mourners felt isolated as they were sent away to the clinician's office to be 'healed'. In this age of the psychological person, the mental health professional and the physician have been assigned the role of 'ritual specialists' for the bereaved, and continue to do so into the twenty-first century. Grief became, and remains, something that, with 'appropriate medicine' or with 'proper treatment', could be expunged as if it were a contagious disease.

Is grief an illness?

The view of grief as an illness permeates into many layers of society (Jacobs 1999; Prigerson and Jacobs 2001) as a continuation of the invisible death described by Ariès (1981). There is an ongoing debate about the value and importance of developing a psychiatric diagnosis called 'traumatic grief' (Jacobs 1999). One argument against establishing a psychiatric disorder for grief is that it encourages containing grief in the doctor's office. Like an illness that can be treated with a little 'penicillin', grief is seen as something that can be diagnosed and cured, thus protecting the community from dealing with the fullness of the way that people's dying changes their world.

Stroebe *et al.* (2001) found that most bereaved people cope well with their grief and find new and constructive ways of dealing with the changes in their lives. I am not ignoring the small percentage of people who, after a death, seem to develop psychiatric problems because of their inability to adapt. It is important to understand their needs, but it is also important to consider that their problem may not be caused by the death itself, but may relate to earlier difficulties in their lives. They may well need professional care and attention. These people, however, are not representative of the general bereaved population.

Robert Lifton (1974) reminds us that we cannot accept death without dealing with mourning, which in its way is a constant reminder that people die. When the pain subsequent to loss is discussed, the emphasis is on how to limit and control it, and ideally, make it go away. The predominant discourse speaks of the need of the bereaved to find closure rather than helping them live through their pain and learn new ways of coping with it. Kleinman and Kleinman (1997) saw the medicalization of suffering creating a problem for society. Friedson (1970: 92) observed: 'A pathology arises when outsiders no longer evaluate the work by rules of logic and knowledge available to all educated men, and when the only legitimate spokesman on an issue relevant to all men must be someone who is officially certified.' Grief is a universal human experience. Everyone needs to be an expert.

The focus on the individual's psyche for gaining an understanding of their grief is reflected in the theories that guided bereavement research for most of the twentieth century. Their major efforts were to prevent the pain and suffering experienced by the bereaved and to minimize the challenge to their well-being associated with the loss. In some ways this created a tension between theory and the actual lives of the bereaved. Mourners often adopted the psychological vocabulary of bereavement and were puzzled when this did not accurately describe their experience or bring them relief in a quick and recognizable way (Silverman 2000).

Bereavement through a twentieth-century lens

Many theories of grief were developed throughout the twentieth century. Stroebe *et al.* (2001) observed that most research focused on the prevention of physical or emotional ill health that was associated with the death of a loved one, and was not guided by an integrative theory of grief. They divided the research into two schools of thought. The first, the psychoanalytical school of thought, evolved from Freud's writings about depression. The second focused on stress theories, examining coping strategies and their impact on mourners' adaptation to their loss.

Psychoanalytical thinking

Most of the earlier research in the twentieth century was conducted by psychiatrists working with mourners who came for psychiatric help. Aspects of depressed behaviour were associated with loss and were seen as the symptomatology of grief, which supported the view of grief as a purely psychological process using the language of medicine and psychology. The focus was on symptoms and outcome. These patients became the psychiatrists' research subjects (Furman 1974; Volkan 1981), and the problems these people presented were then generalized to the larger population of bereaved people. Their problematical behaviours, the pain and confusion following a death, were labelled as symptoms, implying that they were pathological and a sign of illness. It was thought that if the 'correct' form of mourning was followed, these 'symptoms' could be prevented.

Freud's work (1961) had a major impact on this thinking. Freud's early characterization of grief pointed to the necessity of detaching one's memories and expectations from the deceased. He felt that the work of grieving was to let go of the deceased – once emotional investment was removed from the relationship to the deceased, the mourner's emotional energy would be freed for new relationships, as if people could have only one relationship at a time. From his personal letters it is clear that Freud's own experience did not support this view of the trajectory of grief (Silverman and Klass 1996). Nonetheless, his view of how grief ends has dominated most thinking about bereavement in the twentieth century.

In 1944, Lindemann, studying the grief of survivors of a nightclub fire in Boston, identified the three tasks that composed the 'grief work' of these mourners: (i) emancipation from the bond to the deceased; (ii) readjustment to the environment in which the deceased is missing; and (iii) formation of new relationships. He also observed intense guilt in survivors of the fire in which hundreds were killed (Lindemann 1944). These feelings are not unlike those described by Holocaust survivors, who often have difficulty reconciling their own survival with the death that surrounded them (Frankl 1972, 1978; Valent 1994). Today, guilt is invariably looked for in mourners and, when it is not found, the observer often reports that the mourner is repressing or avoiding their feelings. (This is sometimes confused with what some mourners ask in reviewing the circumstances of the death. They ask, 'what if ...?', wondering if somehow they could have prevented the death. This is often a way of trying to get a sense of control in a situation in which there could not have been any. It should not be confused with guilt.)

Lindemann, influenced by Freud, saw grief as ending when the mourner severed his relationship to the deceased. He recognized that the bereaved had to adjust to an environment without the deceased and proposed that the way to do that was to 'let go' of the relationship to the deceased. The focus here was on the mourner's inner emotional life built on their attachment to the deceased.

Bowlby (1980) a psychiatrist with an orientation towards psycho-analysis, was interested in research that would test the validity of psycho-analytical theories of human behaviour current at the time. His work began with studying children who were sent away from their families during the London Blitz in the Second World War, and their reaction to the separation and loss that followed. He published a paper describing the grief he saw in these children at a time of transition (Bowlby 1961). He observed how the children changed emotionally as time distanced them from the loss. He identified an initial period of shock, numbness and disbelief that the loss had occurred, and a gradual acceptance of the impossibility of a reunion. He also observed a phase of yearning and searching, typical of young children, when they tried to find the lost person in order to be reunited with them. He felt that there was a strong tendency to keep a clear visual memory of the deceased, but that the intensity of this memory diminished over time. Following a phase of disorganization and despair, which occurred as the mourner realized that the deceased would not return, came a phase of reorganization in which the bereaved let go of ties to the deceased and established new relationships. With some modification this concept of transition, consistent with what van Gennep described, still applies as we consider the way change works in the grieving process (Silverman 1966, 1986, 2000; Neimeyer 1997).

Bowlby's work had a critical impact on how grief in children was understood, and his research (1980) established that children do grieve. Bowlby described grieving behaviour as observable in all mammals who attach to a primary maternal figure that facilitates their growth and ability to thrive (Osterweis *et al.* 1984). The source of this 'attachment behaviour' emanates, he hypothesized, from an instinctual need to be close to a mothering figure. When this relationship is lost there is sadness, weeping and a threat to the child's sense of well-being. He saw the grief in the children who were evacuated from war-torn London as a form of separation anxiety, which, unlike what happens after an actual death, could be rectified by a reunion with their mothers, or prevented in the first place by limiting the separation. Bowlby's work has been reframed to emphasize the importance of the child's attachment to critical caregivers and how we look at attachment through the life cycle. Researchers of attachment theory talked about types of attachments, but only recently have they begun, again, to talk about issues of loss (Noppe 2000). Bowlby's work puts the emphasis on the relational aspects of grief that are discussed further below.

Furman (1974), like Bowlby a psychiatrist, worked with pre-school children who were in a clinical programme for disturbed children at the time one of their parent's died. Furman identifies three tasks that confront a mourning child: (i) to understand and come to terms with the reality and circumstances of the death; (ii) to mourn; and (iii) to resume and continue their lives. She saw acceptance of the death in these young children coming only after a struggle between disbelief that the death had occurred and confusion about why the deceased was not coming back. Mourning, Furman wrote, involves mastery of this process that comes with loosening ties to the deceased. Mourning ended when the children identified with a part of the deceased, thus allowing them to keep aspects of their lost parent with them for ever. Furman also emphasized the importance of the process of detachment that occurs when the deceased does not come back and children need to withdraw their emotional investment in what is no longer there. Her findings reflect the dilemma faced by clinicians who recognize that people – children and adults – do not detach from the deceased but who were themselves committed to a theory that insisted that this letting go was necessary in order to 'recover'.

Attitudes towards grief that develop in this context emphasize the individual's inner ability to cope. Bereavement is seen not as a communal issue, but as an individual one. Time-limited and contained within the emotional life of the mourner, grief is characterized as something the mourner will get over. Pathology, it was hypothesized, resulted from not grieving as prescribed (Parkes 1996).

Expanding the view of grief

Following on Lindemann's work, the Laboratory of Community Psychiatry at Harvard Medical School, under the direction of Gerald Caplan, sponsored several studies of bereavement. The focus was on the impact of the death on the psychological well-being of these mourners, particularly young widows and widowers (Silverman 1966; Glick *et al.* 1974; Parkes and

Weiss 1983). The voices of sociologists and researchers with a social work and public health background joined the discourse to complement the psychiatric perspective. The initial goal was to learn more about the lives of these widowed people in order to lower the risk of their developing emotional problems that might follow from the death (Silverman 1986; Parkes 1996). This was the goal of the Widow-to-Widow intervention sponsored by the Laboratory (Silverman 1966, 1967, 1986; Silverman et al. 1974). The perspective on grief was expanded by the findings of this research.

A further expansion of the popular view of grief resulted from the work of Lopata (1973). Lopata studied how women's roles and their status as wife in a large urban city defined how they saw themselves and how there were defined by society. She documented the role shifts that took place when they were widowed (Lopata 1973, 1996). If the role of wife is central to a woman's life, what happens when her spouse dies and the role of wife no longer defines her? The focus begins to shift to look at changing relationships, changing roles, in a changing world as a key part of the bereavement process (Silverman 1980, 1986, 2000). Marris (1974) wrote about loss and change introducing other types of losses into the picture. Marris also looked at the nature of change that occurs in the life of the bereaved, describing what he called 'the conservative impulse'. The bereaved, as they came to terms with their new lives, conserved some of the old.

The impact of grief was the subject of a great deal of the research during this period (Osterwies et al. 1984). For the most part, the focus was on identifying how grief negatively affected the physical and mental health of mourners, and interventions were sought that could prevent these outcomes. Factors such as age, role in the family, relationship to the deceased were identified as possibly leading to ill health and problem behaviour. Widowhood was most often the subject of the research. Because of diverse research approaches there is still little consensus about what factors are most critical to which outcome (Stroebe and Schut 2001). Nonetheless, outcome studies have remained one of the key concerns of bereavement research, with much less focus on understanding the grieving process itself.

Bowlby's view of mourning as a time of transition was useful in looking at the grieving process, particularly in understanding the grief of widows and of children (Silverman 1966, 1986; Parkes 1996; Neimeyer 1997). The concept of transition helps to accurately describe what the bereaved go through after the death of a spouse as they adapt to the loss and reorganize their lives, finding new roles for themselves. This approach is also applicable in understanding the impact of the death of a child or the death of a parent. This concept facilitated looking beyond the individual to see grief as a life cycle issue, including family, belief systems and community values (Marris 1974). Parkes (1996) talked about the changes that people experienced in their assumptive worlds, pointing to their need to find a new place for themselves in the world and a new identity. My work elaborated on this from a developmental and relational point of view, focusing on understanding the changing sense of self that results from the loss of a key relationship (Silverman 1988, 2000). Change is seen as an integral part of the grieving process. It becomes possible to talk about the bereaved developing a new narrative about themselves and their place in the world (Silverman 1987, 2000).

A relational paradigm of grief suggests that grief is an interactive process involving multiple mourners and others in the lives of these mourners, highlighting how mutuality and interdependence are expressed in their world views as well as in their daily lives. This focus on relational aspects of grief was propelled, in some ways, by the women's movement. Women observed the importance of relationships in people's lives, and that the goal of development was not independence but interdependence (Miller 1986; Gilligan 1993; Miller and Striver 1997). This shifts the focus from the lone mourner to the world to which they are connected. Relationships with others frame our sense of self and how we live our lives, how we mourn and how we change as a result of this death in our lives.

These relationships frame how we organize and think about death and loss, that is, how we make meaning of this aspect of our lives. As we try to understand the relational world of the mourner, we must include their relationships with the deceased. We are moving towards what I call a relational view of grief – language also used by Weiss (2001) as he described what is lost for the bereaved.

Worden (2001), following on the work of Lindemann and Furman, discussed the tasks to be dealt with if people were to successfully cope with their grief. Rubin (1981, 1996) observed that parents who lost a child followed what he called a two-track model of grief, thus pointing to the importance of the larger social context to the way they coped. He focused on the need to construct a relationship to the deceased, on understanding the personal qualities of the bereaved, and the attitudes and resources in the community in which they lived. Nadeau, in her research, demonstrated the importance of considering grief as a family matter (Rubin *et al.* 2000).

Detachment revisited

The view of grief as something people get over, and the accompanying 'psychologization' of grief, were compatible with the value placed on individual independence and autonomy in western society. Dependency on others was seen as a negative quality (Miller 1986). Relationships with others were viewed instrumentally – in terms of having one's needs met – and the focus of individual development was on separation and indivi-duation. Thus, when a relationship ended, as with a death, it was appropriate to consider how to sever these ties. In this view, by implication, people were seen as having sequential relationships, as if it was possible to have only one close relationship at a time. Different kinds of relationships were not accounted for. Over the years, there were questions raised by researchers as they looked at their data from bereaved families (Silverman and Silverman 1979; Silverman 1986; Klass 1988; Rubin 1992; Silverman *et al.* 1992; Klass *et al.* 1996; Silverman and Klass 1996; Stroebe *et al.* 1996; Walter 1999). The data pointed to how the bereaved remained involved and questioned the merit of the concept of detachment.

Stroebe *et al.* (1996) and Walter (1999) observed that, historically, mourners found ways of continuing their bond with the deceased. For example, Victorian women lived in companionship with the dead for a long time. In that society, the widowed were not expected to let go and get on with their lives, and for most of the twentieth century this was still true. Silverman and Klass (1996), in their review of the recent bereavement research, concluded that there is significant evidence that most bereaved people do not experience the relationship to the deceased as ending at death. Most bereaved people report that letting go of the deceased was not consistent with their experience. The relational and contextual part of their lives needs to be included in order to understand their reactions (Silverman and Klass 1996; Silverman 2000; Klass and Walters 2001). This view challenges the use of the language of recovery, supporting rather the language of accommodation and adaptation.

Stress and coping

Our view of human behaviour is expanding and we consider other 'languages' that helps understand the process of grief. In many ways the language of stress and coping makes it easier to look at grief contextually, that is, focusing on the family, on community resources and on people's learned behaviour in reponding to a death. This view shifts the focus to looking at what people do about their situation. The shift more clearly marks a focus in bereavement work on process, that is, how does mourning unfold, looking not only at an individual mourner but also at their interaction with other mourners, with family and community, at helpful resources, and at values and attitudes prevailing in that society. The focus is less on the intrapsychic aspects of the bereavement process and more on its place in the life cycle and in the daily lives of people (Silverman 2000).

Antonovsky (1979) identified universal stresses – war, murder, hunger and death – which are stressors for everyone. Almost any death, expected or unexpected, can be traumatic, even more so in a society where death is not accepted as a normal part of the life cycle. Lazarus and Folkman (1984), in their studies of stress and coping, not specifically related to bereavement, use the concept of meaning – making to understand how people define and respond to stress. Lazarus and Folkman define stress as the relationship between the person and the environment that is *appraised* by the person as taxing or exceeding their resources. An event becomes stressful when those experiencing it do not know how to define what is happening, or do not know what to do about it and feel that their well-being is in danger. Lazarus and Folkman define coping as the changing thoughts and acts that an individual uses to manage the external or internal demands of stressful situations. Antonovsky (1979) understood that, in many stressful situations, what is overwhelming for some can be transient and fleeting for others. If the individual does not feel threatened, their resources are not taxed, and if their coping strategies are appropriate to deal with the problem, then they will be able to find ways of coping with the situation.

Applying this to bereavement, we see that when someone we care about dies, we are naturally distraught and upset and see our world, at some level, as crumbling. The sense of disarray may come because our way of mapping or coding the world is challenged or not sufficient for the situation (White and Epston 1990; Neimeyer 1998). There may be aspects that the bereaved know how to handle (for example, organizing a funeral or calling people to let them know that the death has occurred), and for those who have accessible mourning rituals these activities can provide some comfort and direction for how to act. The stress may be greater if these traditions are not in place or have no meaning. The lack of funeral and mourning rituals in the community in which the mourner lives may mean that people have little comfort, support or direction as they initially try to deal with the death. There can be a vacuum – even in finding an appropriate way to dispose of the body.

We see that, for many individuals, their resources may be taxed not only by their own ignorance or developmental limitations, but also by the inadequacy of societal resources. A society with an unrealistic understanding of the course of grief can stigmatize the mourner by being afraid of their grief and pulling away from them (Silverman 1969, 2003). The extreme feelings that the mourners experience and which they cannot control, may completely unnerve both themselves and those around them. Greater stress is experienced as they face not only their ongoing emotional responses long after they think they should be finished, but also the fact that they cannot reconstitute their sense of self and their world as before. Few mourners can put their life back in a tidy package in a short period of time, as they are often asked to do (Silverman 1986; Altschul and Altschul 1988; Stroebe *et al.* 1996). Their expectation that they can get over this event in a short time only adds to the sense of disorder. They feel stigmatized and their grief further delegitimized (Silverman 1969, 2003), or, to use Doka's term, they feel disenfranchised (Doka 2001). Richards and Folkman (1997) describe spiritual beliefs and experiences as positively influencing the coping process. The process of grieving opens new doors and can be seen as the impetus for developmental change (Silverman 2000).

It is important to look at how the process of how mourners make meaning, reflects the values and attitudes of the society in which they live and which informs and frames their sense of order and meaning. This concept, of meaning-making, is used in multiple ways. Lazarus and Folkman (1984) used it to describe how people make sense out of (appraise) a problem and decide what to do about it. Neimeyer (1998) writes from a constructivist point of view, viewing human beings as meaning-makers, striving to punctuate, organize and anticipate their engagement with the world by arranging it in themes that express their particular cultures, families and personalities. This is a narrative approach out of which comes a new story, giving meaning to the death and the life once lived (Neimeyer 2001). This directs our thinking away from a single model of grief for all to the importance of family history and culture, as well as the personal qualities of the mourner, in understanding their grief and the direction in which they are going. In some ways this extends Lazarus and Folkman's use of the concept of appraisal.

How people construct meaning also relates to their developmental status, from both cognitive and emotional perspectives (Kegan 1982; Silverman 2000). Both cognitive and emotional development is a process that continues from childhood through old age to death, and is an important factor in how we understand and react to the death. Kegan sees development as a move towards greater complexity and coherence in the way relationships between the self and others are structured, allowing people to move from an egocentric understanding in which the world revolves around them, towards a perspective of greater mutuality. Hence they make new meaning out of their relationships to themselves and to others.

Coping

The concepts of stress and coping go together. The way people cope, that is, respond to the stress they are experiencing, may be more important to their overall morale, social functioning and health than the frequency and severity of the episodes of stress (Rutter 1983). Lazarus and Folkman (1984) define coping as a process of managing the demands of a situation that has been assessed as stressful. Here the application of the way meaning is constructed becomes critical. Coping implies an active grappling with the event and trying to do something about it that depends on how mourners understand what is happening and the resources available in their particular community. Each action sets into motion a process of adaptation extending over time, one effort leading to another. Coping involves how people manage, master, tolerate, reduce and minimize the internal and environmental demands and conflicts. It involves people developing new interpretations of what is happening so that a new story begins to evolve out of their experience (White and Epston 1990). Ideally, in the long run, we look for a flexibility that allows people to respond with a set of responses rather than an enduring trait or style. The focus should be on the process of the management of stress, rather than on mastery. Coping with the death of someone close to us may be a process that continues in different ways for the remainder of our lives.

Grief behaviour – crying and sadness – can be understood as coping efforts, giving voice to the emotions stimulated by the loss. Planning the funeral is another part of the coping process. How people cope at each point in the process creates to some extent the scenario that will follow.

We need to consider the consequences of different coping strategies. It is important to look not only at what is happening to people, but also at the effectiveness of what they *do* with it: does it solve or resolve a particular problem, does it help redefine the situation to make it possible to do something about it, or does it simply create new unsolvable problems? How do people's coping efforts reflect their struggle to give meaning to their situation? There are people who seem to cope more effectively than others, whose meaning-making styles have an almost intuitive flexibility. Antonovsky (1979) identified this ability as 'a sense of coherence'. This coherence affects how people examine and assess the stress. Coherence is tied to the family's openness, to their ability to define the problem and not be defined by it. Folkman (2001) points to the positive impact on mourners of being able to reframe a problem in more positive terms that gave her subjects a sense of control and direction in their activities in a situation where they otherwise had no control, namely over the impending death and the loss it led to in their lives. This ability is also related to their cognitive and emotional development. Effective coping involves giving this stress expression and voice and seeing it as acceptable and expected. It is not always profound actions that make a difference.

Coping that does not seem to remediate or relieve the situation may result from needs that often tax and exceed available resources or that tax the individual's or the family's ability to learn. Thus ineffective coping can become another source of stress. It may be impossible to tease these two concepts – stress and coping – apart completely. It is almost impossible to imagine a stressful situation in which the participants do not do something in response to what is happening. We are always coping – even being frozen in the moment is a reaction.

Lazarus and Folkman (1984) identified two main coping strategies. The first involves problem-solving techniques such as reframing of the problems. This strategy is primarily directed at addressing the issues in the environment or in the individual that pose a threat. This is similar to what White and Epston (1990) call externalizing the problem. Externalizing involves stepping back from the troubling situation to examine it and its meaning.

The second strategy involves regulation of emotions, and in particular the distress that comes as a result of the threat. Denial and distraction are good examples of behaviours that can help achieve a sense of balance, even for the moment. Stroebe and Schut (2001) have reframed these coping modalities that involve regulation of feelings and managing external forces to reflect the experience of people who are dealing with a death. They identify loss-oriented strategies and those that are restoration-oriented. Loss-oriented behaviours help mourners to face their grief and the sense of loss that follows a death. Restorative behaviour involves keeping alive ties to the deceased and the connection to the deceased is encouraged. Stroebe and Schut proposed that, as the bereaved cope, they alternate between these modalities. This is probably true, as most people use more than one way of coping. These ways might include: information gathering, allowing oneself to be supported by others, taking direct action, retreating, cognitively trying to control one's feelings, and finding ways of constructing a relationship to the deceased. People use different responses at different times, in response to different aspects of what they are experiencing. They need to integrate and move between problem-solving strategies and strategies to deal with their feelings. These behaviours are in response not only to what they are experiencing internally but also to the external factors that are a result of the social context in which they are involved. The importance of social support in facilitating effective coping has been documented (Stylianos and Vachon 1993; Folkman 2001). The availability of help that is supportive reflects how a community sees its responsibility to the bereaved and the way caring is expressed.

Another view of grief

We begin to see how bereavement theory has evolved to move beyond focusing on the individual and their private experience. Current thinking is filling some of the gaps in earlier formulations that were insufficient to explain and were incompatible with the experience of bereaved people. The focus has turned to the larger social context in which any given mourner is embedded, with a return to ritual and religious traditions. Other voices needed to be present to see the fullness of what is happening, and that can influence the support and care that is available at this time in people's lives.

I see us coming to a time when grief is seen as a normal, expected period of transition in the life cycle that is associated not only with strong feelings but also with change. All of us who are engaged and attached to others will experience grief. It is important when we speak of grief not to talk about 'them', but about 'us'. Grief and loss touch every person's life. Loss is not simply something that happens to us. Loss is something that we must make sense out of, give meaning to and respond to. When grief may seem to engulf us, we may feel that we have no control over what is happening. Grief is, in fact, something we live through and learn to deal with. Looking at the grieving process, Attig (1996) asks: how do we relearn the world? People who are mourning learn to cope not only with extreme feelings aroused in response to the absence of the deceased, but also with a changed social context. The death can lead to change in many ways. When the deceased is no longer a living presence, we also learn to construct another type of relationship with the deceased. Each aspect of this process influences the others. Thus, when a person is grieving, change is a constant companion. Mourning does not end; as mourners, we do not 'recover'. Rather, we adapt, accommodate and change. All of this results in mourners growing, developing a new perspective on life and how it can and will be lived. All of this may lead to new ways of relating to ourselves and to others. Making an accommodation, in this view, is an active process directed at what, for some, can be seen as a new beginning (Silverman 1988, 2000).

New beginning can be understood on many levels. One way to consider how to understand change is to look at what is lost when someone dies. A relationship is lost; the self that a mourner knew in that relationship is lost and a way of life is lost. This is another way of beginning to look at grief in a relational context, including developing a new relationship with the deceased as well.

When grief is seen as a life cycle event, the larger social and interpersonal context is brought into consideration. People's responses are legitimized by their communities which provide them with support as they learn to live with the pain, accommodate feelings of loss and adjust to the changes in their lives that follow the death. We need to change our question as we look at the pain of the mourner to ask what is right with them, given the circumstances, not what is wrong.

The bereaved do need comfort, support and help as they deal with their grief and find a new direction for their lives. I go back to the research on the role of 'ritual specialist' conducted by Rosenblatt and his colleagues (1976) and ask, who should that helping person be in our postmodern society: grief counsellor, therapist, clergy, family or friends?

The bereaved talk for themselves

The consumer movement has played an important role in how we understand bereavement. Since the late 1960s there has been a growing network of mutual-aid organizations that are run by the bereaved for the bereaved. The pioneers that provided the impetus for these organizations came from my own work with the widowed (Silverman 1966, 1969, 1978) and from England, where bereaved parents organized Compassionate Friends (Stephens 1973) to help each other after a child died. These groups organized, based on the finding that the most helpful person to the newly widowed or newly bereaved parent was another bereaved person. These programmes began to challenge existing views of grief and facilitated another perspective of what grieving people experience (Silverman 1966, 1986, 1988; Klass 1988).

In the USA, the work with the widowed is being carried on in the Widowed Person's Service, a programme of the Association of Retired Persons. Such groups have served as models for other self-help organizations dealing with other kinds of death, such as Mothers Against Drunk Driving. Representatives of these organizations are now included in planning services for the bereaved in many communities nationally, and their influence is impacting our theoretical formulations about the nature of grief.

Conclusion

In part, our difficulty with grief comes from the way human behaviour has been described by the dominant psychological sciences of the past century. We characterize behaviour in linear terms, as if one experience can only lead to one outcome. However, people can rarely be put into a simple cause and effect model (Bruner 1990). We are beginning to recognize the complexity of the human condition and human relationships. In recent decades, we have witnessed a shift to a more realistic view of how we live, with a renewed appreciation of relationships and of the fact that we are very interdependent. It is this care and connection that makes a difference.

We are participating in a changing system, which increasingly looks at the complexity of human relationships and makes invisible deaths impossible. We are moving towards a view of the world that understands that there are things that science can do for us, but that reason can only take us so far on this life journey. We are at a place where former ways of doing things are no longer sufficient. Although new ways have not yet developed, we have to recognize that we cannot control death but we do have choices about how we react to it. Bereavement is not an event that will happen only to others – all of us need to be expert in coping, in making meaning out of death and the grief that will follow.

References

Altschul, S. and Altschul, S. (eds) (1988) *Childhood Bereavement and its Aftermath*, Emotions and Behavior, Monograph 8. New York: International Universities Press.

Antonovsky, A. (1979) *Health, Stress, and Coping*. San Francisco: Jossey-Bass.

Ariès, P. (1981). *The Hour of our Death*. New York: Alfred A. Knopf.

Attig, T. (1996) *How We Grieve: Relearning the World*. New York: Oxford University Press.

Bowlby, J. (1961) Childhood mourning and its implications for psychiatry, *American Journal of Psychiatry*, 118: 481–98.

Bowlby, J. (1980) *Attachment and Loss. Vol. 3, Loss: Sadness and Depression*. New York: Basic Books.

Bruner, J. (1990) *Acts of Meaning*. Cambridge, MA: Harvard University Press.

Charmaz, K. (1994) Conceptual approaches to the study of death, in R. Fulton and R. Bendickson (eds) *Death and Identity*, 3rd edn, pp. 28–79. Philadelphia: The Charles Press.

Doka, K. (ed.) (2001) *Disenfranchised Grief: New Directions, Challenges, and Strategies for Practice*. Chicago: Research Press.

Folkman, S. (2001) Revised coping theory and the process of bereavement, in M. Stroebe, W. Stroebe, R. Hansson and H. Schut (eds) *New Handbook of Bereavement: Consequencess Coping and Care*, pp. 563–84. Washington, DC: American Psychological Association.

Frankl, V. (1972) *The Doctor and the Soul: From Psychotherapy to Logotherapy*. New York: Alfred A. Knopf.

Frankl, V. (1978) *The Unheard Cry for Meaning: Psychotherapy and Humanism*. New York: Simon & Schuster.

Freud, S. (1961) Mourning and melancholia, in J. Strachey (ed. and trans.) *The Standard Edition of the Complete Psychological Works of Sigmund Freud*, Vol. 14, pp. 243–58. New York: Basic Books.

Friedson, E. (1970) Dominant professions, bureaucracy, and client services, in W. Rosengren and M. Lefton (eds) *Organizations and Clients*. Columbus, OH: Merrill.

Fulton, R. (1965) *Death and Identity*. New York: Wiley.

Furman, E. (1974) *A Child's Parent Dies: Studies in Childhood Bereavement*. New Haven, CT: Yale University Press.

Gilligan, C. (1993) *In a Different Voice*. Cambridge, MA: Harvard University Press.

Glick, I.O., Weiss, R.S. and Parkes, C.M. (1974) *The First Year of Bereavement*. New York: John Wiley.

Gorer, G. (1965) *Death, Grief and Mourning in Contemporary Britain*. London: Cresset Press.

Jacobs, S.C. (1999) *Traumatic Grief: Diagnosis, Treatment and Prevention*. Philadelphia, PA: Bruner Mazel.

Kegan, R. (1982) *The Evolving Self*. Cambridge, MA: Harvard University Press.

Klass, D. (1988) *Parental Grief: Solace and Resolution*. New York: Springer.

Klass, D. and Walters, T. (2001) Processes of grief: how bonds are continued, in M.S. Stroebe, R.O. Hansson, W. Stroebe and H. Schut (eds) *Handbook of Bereavement Research: Consequences, Coping and Care*, pp. 431–48. Washington, DC: American Psychological Association.

Klass, D., Silverman, P. R. and Nickman, S. L. (eds) (1996) *Continuing Bonds: New Understandings of Grief*. Bristol, PA: Taylor & Francis.

Kleinman, A. and Kleinman, J. (1997) The appeal of experience; the dismay of images: cultural appropriations of suffering in our times, in A. Kleinman, V. Das and M. Locke (eds) *Social Suffering*, pp. 1–24. Berkeley, CA: University of California Press.

Lazarus, R.S. and Folkman, S. (1984) *Stress, Appraisal, and Coping*. New York: Springer.

Lifton, R.J. (1974) Symbolic immortality, in S.B. Troup and W.A. Greene (eds) *The Patient, Death, and the Family*. New York: Scribners.

Lindemann, E. (1944) Symptomatology and management of acute grief, *American Journal of Psychiatry*, 101: 141–8.

Lopata, H.Z. (1973) *Widowhood in an American City*. Cambridge, MA: Schenkman.

Lopata, H. (1996) *Current Widowhood: Myths and Realities*. Thousand Oaks, CA: Sage.

Marris, P. (1974) *Loss and Change*. London: Routledge & Kegan Paul.

Meyer, J.W. (1988) The social construction of the psychology of childhood: some contemporary processes, in E.M. Hetherington, R.M. Lerner and M. Perlmutter (eds) *Child Development in a Life-span Perspective*, pp. 47–65. Hillsdale, NJ: Lawrence Erlbaum Associates.

Miller, J.B. (1986) *New Psychology of Women*. Boston: Beacon Press.

Miller, J.B. and Stiver, I.P. (1997) *The Healing Connection: How Women Form Relationships in Therapy and in Life*. Boston, MA: Beacon Press.

Neimeyer, R. (1997) Meaning reconstruction and the experience of chronic loss, in K.J. Doka and J. Davidson (eds) *Living with Grief when Illness is Prolonged*, pp. 159–76. Washington, DC: Taylor & Francis.

Neimeyer, R.A. (1998) *Lessons of Loss: A Guide to Coping*. New York: McGraw-Hill.

Neimeyer, R.A. (2001) *Meaning Reconstruction and the Experience of Loss*. Washington, DC: American Psychological Association.

Noppe, I.C. (2000) Beyond broken bonds and broken hearts: the bonding theories of attachment and grief, *Development Review*, 20: 514–38.

Osterweis, M., Solomon, F. and Green, M. (eds) (1984) *Bereavement: Reactions, Consequences and Care*. Washington, DC: National Academy Press.

Parkes, C.M. (1996) *Studies of Grief in Adult Life*, 3rd edn. New York: Routledge.

Parkes, C.M. and Weiss, R.S. (1983) *Recovery from Bereavement*. New York: Basic Books.

Parsons, T. (1994) Death in the western world, in R. Fulton and R. Bendickson (eds) *Death and Identity*, pp. 60–79. Philadelphia: The Charles Press.

Prigerson, H. and Jacobs, S. (2001) Traumatic grief as a distinct disorder: a rational, consensus criteria and a preliminary emperical test. In M.S. Stroebe, R.O. Hansson, W. Stroebe and H. Schut (eds) *Handbook of Bereavement Research: Consequences, Coping and Care*, pp. 613–37. Washington, DC: American Psychological Association.

Richards, T.A. and Folkman, S. (1997) Spiritual aspects of loss at the time of a partner's death from AIDS, *Death Studies*, 21(6): 527–52.

Rosenblatt, P. (2001) A social constructivist perspective on cultural differences in grief, in M.S. Stroebe, R.O. Hansson, W. Stroebe and H. Schut (eds) *Handbook of Bereavement Research: Consequences, Coping and Care*, pp. 285–300. Washington, DC: American Psychological Association.

Rosenblatt, P.C., Walsh, R.P. and Jackson, D.A. (1976) *Grief and Mourning in Cross-cultural Perspective*. New Haven, CT: HRAF Press.

Rubin, S.S. (1981) A two-track model of bereavement: theory and application in research, *American Journal of Orthopsychiatry*, 51: 101–9.

Rubin, S.S. (1992) Adult child loss and the two-track model of bereavement, *Omega*, 24(3): 183–202.

Rubin, S.S. (1996) The wounded family: bereaved parents and the impact of adult child loss, in D. Klass, P.R. Silverman and S.L. Nickman (eds) *Continuing Bonds: New Understandings of Grief*, pp. 217–234. Washington, DC: Taylor & Francis.

Rubin, S., Malkinson, R. and Witztum, E. (2000) An overview of the field of loss, in R. Malkinson, S. Rubin and E. Witztum (eds) *Traumatic and Non-traumatic Loss and Bereavement: Clinical Theory and Practice*, pp. 5–40. Madison, CT: Psychosocial/International Universities Press.

Rutter, M. (1983) Stress, coping and development: some issues and questions, in N. Garmazy and M. Rutter (eds) *Stress, Coping and Development in Children*, p. 1041. New York: McGraw-Hill.

Silverman, P.R. (1966) Services for the widowed during the period of bereavement, *Social Work Practice*. New York: Columbia University Press.

Silverman, P.R. (1967) Services to the widowed: first steps in a program of preventive intervention, *Community Mental Health Journal*, 3: 37–44.

Silverman, P.R. (1969) The Widow-to-Widow program: an experiment in preventive intervention, *Mental Hygiene*, 53: 333–7.

Silverman, P.R. (1978) *Mutual Help Groups: A Guide for Mental Health Workers*, NIMH, DHEW Publication No. (ADM) 78–646, 1978. Washington, DC: US Government Printing Office (reprinted 1980).

Silverman, P.R. (1980) *Mutual Help Groups: Organization and Development*. Beverly Hills, CA: Sage.

Silverman, P.R. (1986) *Widow to Widow*. New York: Springer.

Silverman, P.R. (1987) Widowhood as the next stage in the life cycle, in H.Z. Lopata (ed.) *Widows: North America*. North Carolina: Duke University Press.

Silverman, P.R. (1988) In search of new selves: accommodating to widowhood, in L.A. Bond and B. Wagner (eds) *Families in Transition: Primary Programs that Work*, pp. 200–19. Newbury Park, CA: Sage.

Silverman, P.R. (2000) *Never Too Young to Know: Death in Children's Lives*. New York: Oxford University Press.

Silverman, P.R. (2003) Social support and mutual help for the bereaved, in I.B. Corless, B.B. Germina and M.A. Pittman (eds) *Dying, Death and Bereavement: A Challenge for Living*, 2nd edn, pp. 247–65. New York: Springer.

Silverman, P.R. and Klass, D. (1996) Introduction: What's the problem? in D. Klass, P.R. Silverman and S.L. Nickman (eds) *Continuing Bonds: New Understandings of Grief*, pp. 3–27. Washington, DC: Taylor & Francis.

Silverman, S.M. and Silverman, P.R. (1979) Parent–child communication in widowed families, *American Journal of Psychotherapy*, 33: 429–41.

Silverman, P.R., MacKenzie, D., Pettipas, M. and Wilson, E.W. (eds) (1974) *Helping Each Other in Widowhood*. New York: Health Sciences.

Silverman, P.R., Nickman, S.L. and Worden, J.W. (1992) Detachment revisited: the child's reconstruction of a dead parent, *American Journal of Orthopsychiatry*, 62(4): 493–503.

Stephens, S. (1973) *When Death Comes Home*. New York: Morehouse-Barlow.

Stroebe, M.S. and Schut, H. (2001) Models of coping with bereavement: a review, in M.S. Stroebe, R.O. Hansson, W. Stroebe and H. Schut (eds) *Handbook of*

Bereavement Research: Consequences, Coping, and Care, pp. 375–403. Washington: DC: American Psychological Association.

Stroebe, M., Gergen, M., Gergen, K. and Stroebe, W. (1996). Broken hearts or broken bonds, in D. Klass, P.R. Silverman and S.L. Nickman (eds) *Continuing Bonds: New Understandings of Grief*, pp. 73–86. Washington, DC: Taylor & Francis.

Stroebe, M.S., Hansson, R.O., Stroebe, W. and Schut, H. (2001) Introduction: concepts and issues in contemporary research on bereavement, in M.S. Stroebe, R.O. Hansson, W. Stroebe and H. Schut (eds) *Handbook of Bereavement Research: Consequences, Coping and Care*, pp. 3–22. Washington, DC: American Psychological Association.

Stylianos. S.K. and Vachon, M.L.S. (1993) The role of social support in bereavement, in M. Stroebe, W. Stroebe and R. Hansson (eds) *Bereavement: A Sourcebook of Research and Intervention*, pp. 397–410. Cambridge: Cambridge University Press.

Valent, P. (1994) *Child Survivors of the Holocaust*. New York: Bruner/Routledge.

van Gennep A. (1960) *The Rites of Passage*. Chicago: University of Chicago Press.

Volkan, V.D. (1981) *Linking Objects and Linking Phenomena*. New York: International Universities Press.

Walter, T. (1999) *On Bereavement: The Culture of Grief*. Buckingham: Open University Press.

Weiss, R.S. (2001) Grief, bonds and relationships, in M.S. Stroebe, R.O. Hansson, W. Stroebe and H. Schut (eds) *Handbook of Bereavement Research: Consequences, Coping and Care*, pp. 47–62. Washington, DC: American Psychological Association.

White, M. and Epston, D. (1990) *Narrative Means of Therapeutic Ends*. New York: W.W. Norton.

Worden, J.W. (2001) *Grief Counseling and Grief Therapy: A Handbook for the Mental Health Practitioner*. New York: Springer.

3 | Research in practice

Linda Machin

Traditionally, as in other professions, the practice of palliative and bereavement care was informed by the findings of empirical research, which was based upon the assumption that there is a 'truth' to be discovered by dispassionate and controlled examination of phenomena. The (modernist) belief, which invested science with a unique authority to reveal 'the truth', is challenged by the postmodern perspective which questions the claim 'that we know most about each other when we care the least, when we are cool and distant' (Gergen 1999: 91). The view, therefore, that the practitioner is too subjective to participate in the enterprise of discovery is being over-turned by a new epistemological climate in which clinicians' reported experiences are seen to afford legitimate and important new insights into the human condition. McLeod (1999: 11–12) asserts that 'a reductionist, hypothesis-testing model is fundamentally flawed as an approach to con-structing *practical* knowledge of persons. To carry out research that is relevant to practice, it is necessary that investigations are placed in a con-text of practice.'

This chapter explores three aspects of research, which are central to the concerns of the practitioner in the fields of palliative and bereavement care, using my research illustratively. Those three aspects are:

- The practitioners' relationship with theory as a knowledge base.
- Entering and engaging with the clients' world of grief.
- The organizational role necessary for managing research and ensuring services are grounded in evidence-based practice.

Exploring the bigger picture: the practitioners' relationship with theory as a knowledge base

For all practitioners in palliative and bereavement care, whatever their level of qualification or experience, the 'stories' clients tell are the basis for testing and understanding theory. Do the clients' experiences resonate with what we have been taught and read about the nature of grief? Listening, in addition to its therapeutic purpose, is not simply a process of confirming what academic wisdom has declared to be 'the case', but is a way of recognizing the power of clients to teach, with distinctive and individual insight, what is the nature of grief. As witnesses to clients' human experience, we bear responsibility to give testimony to that experience by promoting its authenticity as a source of knowledge. By attending to the accounts of loss brought by individual clients and considering the broader significance of what we hear, we may discover new ways of looking at loss and bereavement. In this way, we not only test the validity of existing theory but also have the potential to contribute to theory-making.

The clinician, in listening to accounts of the subjective encounter with loss and the process of making sense of it, will hear a range of responses to impending death or bereavement. These different responses are reflected in attitudes to loss and the possible ways of finding a new sense of coherence within the chaos of grief. A search for 'a sense of coherence' (Antonovsky 1988) is an essential part of the cognitive process of managing grief and reorientation to the consequences of loss. As practitioners, we listen to individual stories of grief and are witness to people's attempts to revise their 'assumptive world' (Parkes 1996) and review previous 'structures of meaning' (Marris 1974). However, what we hear from individual clients is not simply an account of an inner world of feeling and meaning-making, but a narrative, which reveals a structured way of telling the 'story' of experience, reflecting a historically and culturally specific perspective (Burr 1995). As a practitioner and researcher, I wondered, are there any patterns in these diverse responses to loss? What is the relationship between 'this' client and the wider social discourse, which has shaped their perspective?

I wanted to know, as a practitioner, how existing theory might help in answering these questions. Attachment theory has been influential in shaping our understanding of grief (Bowlby 1980). It suggests that variation in attachment styles, which are the consequence of experiences in significant early relationships, provide a theoretical rationale for understanding the range of differences in coping with separation and loss. The definition of these styles and their manifestation, described by Ainsworth *et al.* (1978) as secure attachment, ambivalent attachment and avoidant attachment, provided a theoretical reference point for clinical observation.

In moving beyond theoretical descriptions of the nature of grief into the immediate context of practice, concepts of 'risk' in grief (Parkes and Weiss

1983; Rando 1992; Parkes 1996) have provided a theoretical base upon which practitioners might determine the need for therapeutic intervention. The concept of risk has been particularly important in the assessment of bereavement need in palliative care settings. Risk theory suggests that the degree of resilience in the mourner and the nature of the loss sustained are factors which will predict low risk (normal grief) or high risk (pathological variations of grief). In some circumstances, the risk classification may be a helpful guide to grieving needs, but in my work, it was by no means universally indicative of problematic grief. For some people, a bereavement which was predictable and timely (for example that of an older person after a period of health deterioration), seemed to produce overwhelming grief, whereas in other circumstances someone might respond with equanimity to the loss, for example, of a young person in an accident. What was my own work telling me and how did it provide a link between (existing and possibly new) theory and practice?

Embedded in the accounts of personal histories of relationships and acquired belief about self and the world, I heard highly individual reactions to loss (Machin 1980, 2001). Nevertheless, within those individual stories of grief I observed three broadly different grief reactions or discourses. These differences were characterized as:

- Overwhelmed, where people were deeply sunk into the distress of grief.
- Balanced, where people were able to face the emotional and practical consequences of loss with equilibrium.
- Controlled, where people demonstrated a need to manage their emotions and retain a primary focus upon ongoing life demands.

I combined these notions of difference into a theoretical framework (the Range of Response to Loss framework, RRL) which provided a conceptual structure within which it was proposed that an 'overwhelmed', 'balanced' or 'controlled' discourse might be heard and expressed (see Figure 3.1).

This structure for looking at grief suggested that the 'storied world' (Sarbin 1986) of loss, which has been shaped by cultural and social ways of understanding the nature and impact of grief, would be evident in the narrative account of death, dying or bereavement heard in practice.

These categories of difference were conceptualized in the language brought by clients to therapy. They resonate with, and provide a particular practice focus on, other theoretical propositions (for example attachment theory, Ainsworth *et al.* 1978; Bowlby 1980), but particularly that of the contemporary dual process model of grief (Stroebe and Schut 1999 – see Figure 3.2). This latter theory has challenged the traditional psychodynamic view of grief with its emphasis upon an introverted, emotion-focused process believed to be essential for the satisfactory resolution of grief (Freud 1917; Bowlby 1980). By giving recognition to the tasks of restoration,

Figure 3.1 The RRL framework

| | Range of Response to Loss (RRL) | | |
	1 Overwhelmed	2 Balanced	3 Controlled
Perspectives on loss, i.e. discourse on loss	An experience of loss can be overwhelming	An experience of loss can be met with **equanimity/balance**	An experience of loss can be **subdued/controlled**
Personal identification with a loss perspective	'I cannot deal with loss and change'	'I can face loss and change'	'I can control loss and change'
A personal narrative account of an experience of loss	'This loss has taken over my life'	'Although it is difficult, I know I have the strength, and other people's support, to help me through this loss'	'If I divert from this loss I can manage perfectly well'
A response to other people's loss within the discourse framework	'I have suffered much more than you have'	'I recognize your pain and hope that, like me, you will find the support you need'	'Don't trouble me with your loss. You need to get on with life, as I have'

Figure 3.2 Conceptual comparisons among the RRL framework, attachment style and the dual process model

Range of Response to Loss (RRL)	Group 1 Overwhelmed by loss	Group 2 Balanced approach to loss	Group 3 Control of loss
Ainsworth *et al.* 'attachment' style (1978)	Anxious/ambivalent attachment	Secure attachment	Avoidant attachment
Stroebe and Schut dual process model (1999)	Loss orientation	← oscillation →	Restoration orientation

which embrace the cognitive and social aspects of loss reaction, Stroebe and Schut (1999) have given new credence to wider expressions of grief. They have provided a comprehensive account of grief and its individual complexity as people 'oscillate' between loss (i.e. focus on grief work) and restoration (i.e. focus on avoidance, doing other things).

How might the validity of the proposed discourses in the RRL framework be tested? Attitudes link experience with action and reaction (Eagly and Chaiken 1993) and are revealed in the accounts of grief brought to therapy. For this reason an attitudinal scale seemed to provide the potential for accessing and exploring different responses to loss. The Adult Attitude to Grief scale (AAG scale – see Appendix 1) was devised for and used in Machin's study (Machin 2001). It was based upon nine attitudinal statements, which reflected the proposed categories of loss response: overwhelmed, balanced and controlled. Three statements were associated with each of the categories: 2, 5, 7 reflected the overwhelmed perspective; 1, 3, 9 linked with the balanced perspective; and 4, 6, 8 demonstrated a controlled loss response.

The validity of the AAG scale as a measure used to distinguish three broad differences in loss response, identified in the RRL framework, was obtained from quantitative analysis of data in a study sample of 94 people seeking counselling support in their bereavement (Machin 2001). Each person completed the AAG scale on two occasions, separated by six months. Factor analysis confirmed that the AAG scale provided a good measure of the three proposed categories of overwhelmed, balanced and controlled. Further analysis showed that, whereas the 'balanced' and 'controlled' responses showed predictable consistency over time, this was not the case with the 'overwhelmed' responses. The 'overwhelmed' statements captured something of the transitional qualities of grief, specifically difficulty in detaching focus from the deceased (Leiden Detachment scale – see Cleiren 1991). For the 'balanced' items there was no evidence of association with distress factors, such as depression (Beck *et al.* 1961). Increased age was predictive of a controlled response to the AAG items.

While supporting the notion of broad categories of difference contained in the RRL framework, the AAG scale emerged as a more powerful tool for exploring the complex characteristics of grief in individuals. This provided a new theoretical articulation of grief, recognizable in practice, as clients endeavour to manage the overwhelming aspects of unbidden anguish, attempt to establish control in an out-of-control situation, and search for a balance between feelings, thoughts and action. In a climate in which theory is giving greater emphasis to the need to understand individual grieving processes, this seemed an important development.

Work within palliative and bereavement care can provide the richest possible setting for understanding the phenomenon of grief. The stories of loss which we hear will resonate with accepted theories of grief, but we need to be alert to the theoretical principles which may be drawn from our own engagement with dying and bereaved people.

Meeting with mourning – entering and engaging with the client's world of grief

Following the research (Machin 2001) in which the AAG scale was shown to have the potential to examine the spectrum of emotional and cognitive grief perspectives in individual clients, a new research question emerged. How might the AAG scale facilitate the telling of the individual 'story' of loss and provide the clinician with a profile of grief which might guide the therapeutic process?

To answer this question, a study of the AAG scale in practice was undertaken within a Clinical Psychology service which takes referrals from hospital and community-based professionals (Machin and Spall 2004). Action research was the method used in the study (also called the Human Inquiry method), which is a cyclical process where hypotheses are considered, tested, reviewed and revised by a group of practitioners who are also the researchers (Reason 1988). In this approach, research is integrated within the existing therapeutic process and subject to the conventions regulating ethical practice. For the practitioner, the merit of this method is that its reflective nature makes use of existing expertise, while promoting new ways of thinking about clients and the work with them.

The year-long, three-phase study, consisting of action, reflection and revision, produced interesting evidence of the efficacy of the AAG scale as a tool to facilitate therapeutic dialogue. It provided an entrance into the clients' grief and their perspectives on how to manage distress. There was an uncovering of key concerns and issues which flowed very naturally from the attitudinal items and the themes associated with them. With some clients this provided insight into factors of their grief which had not been revealed by other therapeutic methods. The AAG scale proved to be an appropriate and comfortable tool for both the clinician and the clients. While the scale was easy to administer (it is not a long instrument), it was necessary to be alert to possible negative reactions by clients. In this small sample ($N = 15$) there were no contraindications. However, the need to be sensitive to the use of the AAG scale was always recognized. Practitioners used their judgement about circumstances in which intellectual/cognitive approaches to exploring distress might be inappropriate (for example where the age, physical or mental health/capacity of the client required a simple, practical focus).

A practice consequence of the study was the development of a protocol for the clinical use of the AAG scale (see Figure 3.3).

Figure 3.3   A therapeutic process for mapping grief using the AAG scale

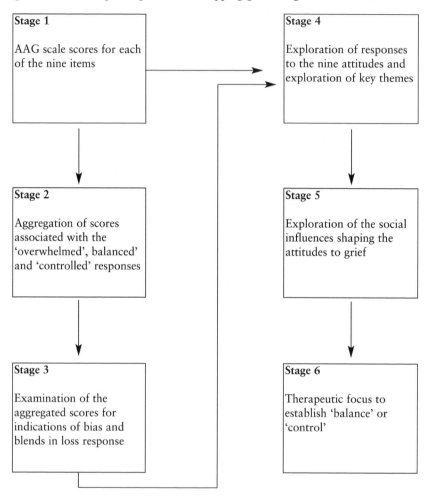

This six-stage protocol for 'mapping grief' began with three quantitative elements.

Stage 1. The client completes the scores for each of the nine items on the questionnaire. This may be done alone or with the assistance of the practitioner.

Stage 2. The scores for each of the three categories (overwhelmed, balanced and controlled) are aggregated. The lowest possible aggregated score within each category is 3; the highest is 15. A low score indicates strong agreement and a high score indicates strong disagreement.

Stage 3. Detailed appraisal is necessary as scores are examined to provide a unique profile of the client's loss response.

• Examination of the aggregated scores to see if there is a general directional *bias* towards an 'overwhelmed', 'balanced' or 'controlled' response to loss.
• Exploration of the scores for each item on the AAG scale in order to see how different attitudes coexist (i.e. recognizing the *blends* of response spanning the 'overwhelmed', 'balanced' and 'controlled' statements).
• Appraisal of the nature and extent of attitudinal *consistency and inconsistency* within the responses made to the items across the whole AAG scale (i.e. are there attitudinal contradictions?)

These three stages can be usefully repeated at points throughout the therapeutic process. This indicates the direction of change (if any), which is helpful to both the practitioner and the client. The repeat use of the AAG scale might also be employed as an outcome measure.

Figure 3.4 gives a case example of the way in which stages 1–3 of the protocol were used in the 2003 study.

Stages 4–6 provide qualitative focus on the narrative voice of the client. (Practitioners may choose to use the AAG scale but retain a largely qualitative approach by moving from stage 1 to stage 4.)

Stage 4. The client is invited to elaborate on their responses to each of the nine items in the AAG scale and to explore pertinent issues prompted by them. Some broad themes associated with each of the nine attitudinal statements may also widen the cues to the loss narrative:

• The ability to confront loss
• The intrusion of grief
• A sense of one's own resourcefulness
• A need to appear all right
• The persistence of grief
• The need to control
• A sense that everything is changed
• The need to divert
• The possibility of a positive outcome

Stage 5. The grief perspective of clients reflects both their wider social context (including family, and religious and cultural influences) and the history of losses which they have experienced. It is important to give full recognition to the social background against which attitudes to grief are shaped. Some attitudes will have come from (been learned from) other people – 'What we say on any occasion – even when we are convinced that it is "my belief" – is often reflecting a voice we have appropriated from

Figure 3.4   A case example of the quantitative use of the AAG scale

Factor	AAG items	Score T1	Agg. score	Score T2	Agg. score	Score T3	Agg. score
Over-whelmed	2	1		2		2	
	5	1	3	1	5	4	8
	7	1		2		2	
Balanced	1	4		4		2	
	3	2	10	2	8	1	5
	9	4		2		2	
Controlled	4	1		2		1	
	6	1	3	2	6	2	4
	8	1		2		1	

Rob was a widower who was considered to be a suicide risk. He had difficulty in accepting that his wife was dead and described himself as 'being in a dream'. In the face of unrelenting denial and heightened psychological vulnerability, the task, for the practitioner, of engaging with the internal and external reality of the client was challenging. The AAG scale was used on three occasions during the therapeutic process, to help Rob explore his grief and to move beyond the initial block in facing the emotional and social consequences of his bereavement.

Time 1 (T1) – The strong agreement (aggregated score 3) with both the 'overwhelmed' and the 'controlled' statements indicated a tension between Rob's actual (overwhelming) feelings and his aspirations to manage (control) his grief. This was evident in the clinical manifestation of his distress and his disagreement (individual score 4) with two of the 'balanced' statements, which indicated a negative view of his own capacity to handle grief.

Time 2 (T2) – There was a clear reduction in the strength of his 'overwhelming' feelings (aggregated score 5) and his need for 'control' (aggregated score 6), matched by a greater sense of his own resourcefulness ('balance' – aggregated score 8). This change in scores helps to show the movement in Rob's perspectives, which was also evident in the reduction in the psychological distress seen by his therapist. At this stage it was useful for the therapist to explore item/statement 5 (score 1) and item/statement 1 (score 4) as the two items on the scale which produced different and opposite responses.

Time 3 (T3) – 'Control' had become the strongest attitudinal bias, there was a reduction in the strength of his 'overwhelming' feeling and greater association with the 'balanced' statements. Rob had moved to a position where he could feel more in control through having been helped to engage with his own strengths and resourcefulness (the perspectives contained in the 'balanced' items/statements).

another' (Gergen 1999: 174); some attitudes will have developed as a result of an earlier experience of loss; some attitudes may reflect the current expectation of other people; or attitudes may be a mix of these factors. The social context of grieving not only influences attitudes and behaviours towards loss but also is the arena in which collective social responses might be made (for example, rituals) and within which support may be provided (or not). Significant others might usefully complete the AAG scale in order to explore the grieving social dynamic within a family (for example, the extent to which a wife may be grieving the losses arising from her husband's terminal illness, where the husband is the client).

Stage 6. The 'story' of grief, which will have emerged through the narrative account of loss, facilitated by the cues provided by the AAG scale, will have provided a picture of the client and of their experience of loss/bereavement. A desired therapeutic objective might be defined as one in which there is increased capacity to deal with the emotional distress of loss and a greater facility to manage the cognitive and social consequences of it; a 'balanced' perspective (Shaver and Tancredy 2001). However, the client will also be giving indications about the ways in which they would like to respond to a changed life situation and possible desired outcomes. For some clients there may be a more limited objective: that of being in 'control'. This is some-times seen as safer than dealing introspectively with grief. Whichever objective is set, it needs to be consistent with the client's own aspirations for change. At the very least the client is likely to want to be able to address (or subdue) the 'overwhelming' aspects of the distress caused by grief. A wide therapeutic repertoire is necessary to achieve these objectives in a way which is sensitive to the highly individual nature of grief.

Action research is a dialogic process of finding out, in which the expertise of the practitioner has a valued role in exploring links between theory and practice. The practitioner's engagement with the client's grief is powerfully exposed to review, new insight and modification. As exemplified in the study described here, action research provided the impetus for a develop-ment in practice, a new method of entering and engaging with the client's world of grief.

Creating a research climate – the organizational concern for evidence-based practice

So far this chapter has examined the way in which a critically reflexive approach to practice can contribute to the development of new ways of thinking about theory. It has also provided an example of a method of accessing clients' stories of loss and initiating a therapeutic process, which attends to the individual nature of grief. However, this demands that the organizational settings in which practice occurs must be capable of responding to research opportunities and responsibilities. It requires an understanding of the nature and purpose of research in addressing needs within palliative and bereavement care, and appropriate organizational policies and strategies to sustain it.

Whereas in statutory care, especially health care, there are well-established structures for the oversight and maintenance of standards in research, in voluntary care settings a new research function may have to be developed. The concern to deliver a quality service requires an organizational structure, which embraces a research focus. This aspect of an organization's function should be to set aims and objectives to determine a research policy, to oversee research proposals, to monitor and supervise research in progress, and to integrate findings into practice. Medical ethics committees are central to the research function within health care. This setting, centring as it does upon medical investigations, drug trials and so on, has favoured the use of randomized controlled trials (RCTs), which assign clients, usually large numbers, to different treatments randomly. The RCT approach is seen to have a methodological rigour and scientific credibility, absent from qualitative research undertaken by practitioners in the allied fields of psychosocial care. Tension can exist, therefore, between traditional positivist research and the newer demands for methodological pluralism. For practitioners, the use of clients as research subjects brings a particular tension. The management of the tension between practice and research places significant responsibility upon an organization, but this should not be avoided by neglecting the ongoing quest for new insight and more effective ways of working with the dying and the bereaved (Parkes 1995; Stroebe *et al.* 2001). Developing a research culture in which there is commitment to its place within the total enterprise of palliative and bereavement care is vital.

The requirement for research is driven not least by a need to respond to standards set by professional groups, training institutions, funding bodies, public 'watchdog' organizations, and service users, all of whom demand that practice be based upon assured quality. Such assurance is seen in contemporary professional settings as 'evidence-based practice', in which the efficacy and competence of therapeutic intervention are thoroughly tested, and the conclusions used to provide demonstrable guides to good practice. The investigative, enquiring and testing activities of research provide the partnership necessary to ensure that practice is competently, appropriately and ethically undertaken. The notion of evidence-based practice firmly implies the integration of research in practice. McLeod (1994: 10) asserts this (with reference to counselling): 'Research is a component of all competent practice. It is not possible to be a good counsellor without possessing a spirit of openness to inquiry. Good research in the domain of counselling and psychotherapy always exists in an alive dialectic relationship with practice.'

No single research method addresses all aspects of enquiry, monitoring and evaluation (McLeod 1994). In medical settings, this demands a move away from RCTs as the only form of research and one which is ill suited to studies in psychosocial care. Organizations and individuals need to recognize that several approaches will contribute to a repertoire of practice-focused research in the fields of palliative and bereavement care.

All organizations keep records of their service users and the work which has been undertaken with them, whether this is medical notes or therapeutic case records. This data provides important demographic information about the scope of practice within an organization. Not only can it be used for descriptive and quantitative accounts of practice, but it can also be examined more closely to identify, for example, the range of service provision, the gaps in service provision, areas for service development and areas for future research.

Appraising the efficacy of service provision is part of the professional supervisory function (by attending to individual client care, supervisors and carers can jointly consider the actual and potential skills necessary to meet the need of a service user). At an organizational level, overall scrutiny of the efficacy of its own service provision needs to be pursued by systematic outcome methods. This needs to be undertaken by evaluating both the process and the outcome of professional intervention at the end of therapy. By looking at the theoretical premises upon which care was provided, practitioners can participate in appraising the extent to which goals were met. Specific outcome measures are also important, and while there has been comparatively little work done to develop such measures, the most recent overview of research into practice efficacy believes that the time is right for a more rigorous approach to the study of the effects of bereavement intervention (Schut et al. 2001). The Adult Attitude to Grief scale is a tool which in repeat use has demonstrated the capacity to record change, and might, therefore, be considered as an outcome measure. Clearly, more research is needed to test this possibility.

A growing element within outcome studies is the attention to clients' own satisfaction with a service and their perspective on the efficacy of the help they have received (Leiper and Field 1993; Machin and Pierce 1996). This is another way in which the voice of those who grieve is being legitimized. (Chapter 6 of this book looks more closely at this aspect of research.)

In the sphere of palliative and bereavement care, new attention has been given to client groups underusing services (for example, members of ethnic minority groups) and those perceived to be a particularly vulnerable client group (for example, children, people with a learning disability). Developing new areas of practice can be daunting, but a small-scale trial or 'pilot' is a useful way of undertaking a manageable piece of research. Action research, already discussed in this chapter, is where the practitioner moves between a therapeutic role and that of investigator, testing out new ideas and establishing theories, which in turn shape their practice. A small-scale trial can be used to focus on the needs of a particular client group, the skills required to work effectively with them, procedures for appropriate assessment, and the accumulated learning for dissemination to other practitioners (Machin 1993). Pilot studies can also be used to test therapeutic materials such as pictures, booklets and practitioner manuals to assist in the consistent and confident therapeutic engagement with clients (Read 2001).

Individual practitioners raise research agendas from a desire to discover something which is of interest in their own work or is part of study for a qualification, such as a master's degree. Organizations need both to foster and to monitor such small-scale studies, sharing and encouraging the enthusiasm which individuals often bring to the work. They do, however, have the responsibility to provide ongoing ethical guidance and supervision.

Organizations need a research-focused forum in which the priorities for research, the conduct of it and the integration of new learning into practice can be determined. Medical settings and voluntary groups will operate differently, but by having a visible commitment to new ways of understanding and new ways of providing care, the integration of research into practice contributes to a dynamic and evidence-based culture.

Conclusion

This chapter has looked at the relationship between research and practice in the spheres of theory-making, engagement with clients' grief, and organizational responsibility for evidence-based practice. As practitioners we are important players in the quest for 'knowing'. Tradition and traditional methods of research may have relegated us to the sidelines, but it is crucial that we give testimony to the voice of our clients in a climate which is less challenging of our right to do so. 'The hierarchy of theory over practice is replaced by a level field: we are all practitioners in the creation of cultural life. Further, because we are "all in it together" we are invited to share, to place practices of theory and action into collaborative, catalytic and creative relationship' (Gergen 1999: 167). As practitioners we must rise to the challenge to use our own source of knowing for the good of the dying and bereaved we serve.

References

Ainsworth, M.D.S., Blehar, M.C., Waters, E. and Wall, S. (1978) *Patterns of Attachment: A Psychological Study of the Strange Situation*. Hillsdale, NJ: Erlbaum.

Antonovsky, A. (1988) *Unraveling the Mystery of Health: How People Manage*

Stress and Stay Well. San Francisco: Jossey-Bass.

Beck, A.T., Ward, C.H., Mendelson, M., Mock, J.E. and Erbaugh, J. (1961) An inventory for measuring depression, *Archives of General Psychiatry*, 4: 561–71.

Bowlby, J. (1980) *Attachment and Loss. Vol. 3, Loss: Sadness and Depression*. Harmondsworth: Penguin.

Burr, V. (1995) *An Introduction to Social Constructionism*. London: Routledge.

Cleiren, M. (1991) *Bereavement and Adaptation: A Comparative Study of the Aftermath of Death*. Washington, DC: Hemisphere.

Eagly, A.H. and Chaiken, S. (1993) *The Psychology of Attitudes*. Fort Worth, TX: Harcourt Brace Jovanovich.

Freud, S. (1917) Mourning and melancholia, in *Sigmund Freud: Collected Papers*, Vol. 4. New York: Basic Books.

Gergen, K.J. (1999) *An Invitation to Social Construction*. London: Sage.

Leiper, R. and Field, V. (eds) (1993) *Counting for Something in Mental Health Services: Effective User Feedback*. Aldershot: Avebury.

McLeod, J. (1994) *Doing Counselling Research*. London: Sage.

McLeod, J. (1999) *Practitioner Research in Counselling*. London: Sage.

Machin, L. (1980) *Living with Loss*. Research report for the Lichfield Diocesan Board for Social Responsibility, UK.

Machin, L. (1993) *Working with Young People in a Loss Situation*. Harlow: Longman.

Machin, L. (2001) Exploring a framework for understanding the range of response to loss: a study of clients receiving bereavement counselling. PhD thesis, Keele University, UK.

Machin, L. and Pierce, G. (1996) *Research: A Route to Good Practice*. Keele: Keele University Centre for Counselling Studies.

Machin, L. and Spall, R. (2004) Mapping grief: a study in practice, *Counselling and Psychotherapy Research*, 4(1): 9–17.

Marris, P. (1974) *Loss and Change*. London: Routledge & Kegan Paul.

Parkes, C.M. (1995) Guidelines for conducting ethical research, *Death Studies*, 19: 171–81.

Parkes, C.M. (1996) *Bereavement: Studies of Grief in Adult Life*. London: Routledge.

Parkes, C.M. and Weiss, R.S. (1983) *Recovery from Bereavement*. New York: Basic Books.

Rando, T.A. (1992) The increasing prevalence of complicated mourning: the onslaught is just beginning, *Omega*, 26(1): 43–59.

Read, S. (2001) A year in the life of a bereavement and counselling support service for people with a learning disability, *Journal of Learning Disability*, 15(1): 19–33.

Reason, P. (ed.) (1988) *Human Inquiry in Action: Developments in New Paradigm Research*. London: Sage.

Sarbin, T.R. (1986) The narrative as a root metaphor for psychology, in T.R. Sabin (ed.) *Narrative Psychology: The Storied Nature of Human Conduct*. New York: Praeger.

Schut, H., Stroebe, M.S., Van Den Bout, J. and Terheggen, M. (2001) The efficacy of bereavement interventions: determining who benefits, in M.S. Stroebe, R.O. Hansson, W. Stroebe and H. Schut (eds) *Handbook of Bereavement Research*. Washington, DC: American Psychological Association.

Shaver, P.R. and Tancredy, C.M. (2001) Emotion, attachment and bereavement: a conceptual commentary, in M.S. Stroebe, R.O. Hansson, W. Stroebe and H. Schut (eds) *Handbook of Bereavement Research*. Washington, DC: American Psychological Association.

Stroebe, M. and Schut, H. (1999) The dual process model of coping with bereavement: rationale and description, *Death Studies*, 23: 197–224.

Stroebe, M., Hansson, R.O., Stroebe, W. and Schut, H. (2001) Future directions for breavement research, in M.S. Stroebe, R.O. Hansson, W. Stroebe and H. Schut (eds) *Handbook of Bereavement Research*. Washington, DC: American Psychological Association.

Appendix 1: Adult Attitude of Grief scale

Indicate your response to the attitudes expressed in the following statements:

Strongly agree / agree / neither agree nor disagree / disagree / strongly disagree

| 1 | 2 | 3 | 4 | 5 |

1. I feel able to face the pain which comes with loss.

| 1 | 2 | 3 | 4 | 5 |

2. For me, it is difficult to switch off thoughts about the person I have lost.

| 1 | 2 | 3 | 4 | 5 |

3. I feel very aware of my inner strength when faced with grief.

| 1 | 2 | 3 | 4 | 5 |

4. I believe that I must be brave in the face of loss.

| 1 | 2 | 3 | 4 | 5 |

5. I feel that I will always carry the pain of grief with me.

| 1 | 2 | 3 | 4 | 5 |

6. For me, it is important to keep my grief under control.

| 1 | 2 | 3 | 4 | 5 |

7. I believe that nothing will ever be the same after an important loss.

| 1 | 2 | 3 | 4 | 5 |

8. I think it's best just to get on with life after a loss.

| 1 | 2 | 3 | 4 | 5 |

9. It may not always feel like it but I do come through the experience of grief.

| 1 | 2 | 3 | 4 | 5 |

Jenny Altschuler

Adaptation to a medical diagnosis demands a radical reorganization of individual and family life. Drawing on clinical experience, this chapter focuses on loss and resilience in exploring the way in which families negotiate the impact of illness on their everyday lives. Although 'family' will be used, this term evokes different images for us all. Eurocentric literature regards the family as the primary social group into which we are born, and on whom we depend for nurturance and socialization. However, this is not applicable for all: changes in patterns of cohabitation, increased divorce rates and the introduction of new family forms by immigrant communities, have widened the meaning of family life in the UK. So too, images of 'the family' have to alter in facing illness and death. For communities where high proportions of people have been affected and infected by HIV and AIDS, such as the East African community in London, definitions of family and parenting have had to alter to embrace the reality that nurturance and socialization of young children are often provided by older siblings, extended family, friends or foster family (Kaniuk 1997; Miah 2004).

Confronted with a chronic or life-threatening illness, each family member has to redefine their expectations of themselves and their relationships to one another. This is not unique to illness. We all negotiate multiple contradictions in everyday life: some experiences enhance our sense of coherence whereas others are more challenging, requiring a profound redefinition of who we are. Adults and children who have previously adjusted well, may struggle enormously in the face of illness. Others find they have resources they were unaware of, that illness enables them to find a new way of thinking about themselves and relating to one another. Indeed, current research focused on a range of transitions, such as illness, divorce, death and war-related trauma, has moved from trying to understand risk factors to looking at mechanisms mediating psychological risk, reducing the impact of adversity and probability of negative chain reactions (Jenkins and Smith 1990; Garmezy and Masten 1994; Ayalon 1998; Rutter 1999). What appears crucial to dealing with traumatic transitions is access to confirming relationships, the opportunity for self-reflection, and some area of competence that enables us to develop and redefine a sense of self-esteem.

This research highlights that the way we negotiate moving between being defined as healthy to being defined as ill is not self-determined but influenced by the ideas of family members, professionals and the wider social context in which we live. Distinctions between health and illness are far from clear: research highlights considerable variability in diagnosis, treatment and health-seeking behaviour across location, social class, cultural, gendered and racialized groupings (Radley 1994; Kelleher and Hillier 1996; Dwivedi 1999). Indeed, increased migration to the UK has highlighted the extent to which illness is culturally constructed, influencing decisions about caring for oneself and others, expectations of official institutions and the readiness to accept help (Krause *et al.* 1990; Krause 1998; Altschuler 2002).

The very words used to denote an illness may affect how we see ourselves: Sontag (1991) illustrates how the terms 'cancer' and 'AIDS' not only denote medical conditions but have become 'lurid' metaphors for what is shameful or avoidable in life. All too often, the stigma of AIDS locks adults and children in a private world of secrets and shame. Even in southern Africa, where the condition is highly prevalent, it is difficult to share or make sense of what is happening for fear of exposing others to further humiliation and alienation. Paradoxically, recognizing the role that psychological factors may play in influencing health has added to the burden of being ill: the suggestion that one can 'fight' cancer with the correct mental attitude has meant that a recurrence of cancer is seen by many as a personal failure.

Systems theory offers a useful framework for conceptualizing the experience of illness for families and health professionals alike. It places illness and loss within the context of interpersonal relationships, outlining that:

- any organization, be this a family or health care unit, can be defined as a system in which the sum of the parts is different from that of the whole;
- systems have a fragile balance: change to any one part of a system affects the rest of the system;
- difficulties are more likely to arise at times of transition: entrances and exits, such as changes in staffing, a patient dying, and changes to existing hierarchy and alliances, alter the structure of a system;
- there is a connection between beliefs and behaviour: beliefs about loss, parenting and blame influence both experiences and behaviour;

- what we observe around us can be understood in different ways: the beliefs, expectations and experience of the person defined as ill may be very different from those of the health professional or family members;
- an observer is inevitably part of the system being observed: any analysis of the people with whom we work cannot be separated from the meaning of the experiences for ourselves.

Experiences vary and are dependent on the nature of the condition itself, treatment, and individual and family factors. A medical diagnosis may mean having to live with restricted activity, attending numerous appointments, participating in painful and tiring medical procedures, and dependence on others. Both children and adults may have to undergo painful or scarring treatment, take large doses of medication or spend long periods attached to machinery, altering their body image and sense of autonomy. This requires the patient to balance fear and uncertainty, both their own and that of the people upon whom they are temporarily or permanently dependent. Faced with cancer or multiple sclerosis, ill parents may find themselves having to prioritize their own needs, challenging core beliefs about parenting. One mother expressed this as competing with her baby, stating: 'I feel, I mean it feels like this, ... there's two things that are competing, that's the cancer and there's the baby.'

What does loss mean for families facing illness?

When someone is diagnosed as seriously ill, each member of the family tends to move between grief and hope, trying to find some connection between past and future life. We have different ways of responding to this: some deny what is happening, retaining as much pre-illness identity as possible, whereas others prefer to prepare for each eventuality; some find hope in spirituality, while others focus energy on self-help healing programmes, such as diet and exercise. Initially, denial may be adaptive, a way of managing chaos and confusion. However, if retained in terminal phases, it can become problematical, isolating family members just when mutual support is most needed.

Often, grieving is most intense as the permanence of the situation is accepted. However, it would be inappropriate to focus purely on suffering: illness provides a chance to experience oneself and others in a different way, to heal past wounds, experience being cared for and to reassess personal and shared goals. A growth in self-worth can evolve from caring for one another, learning to value what others can give, developing compassion and delaying gratification.

Perhaps what is most complex is how family members face the difference and imbalance imposed by illness. Ill and healthy members face different futures, and there may be disparities in how they balance hope with acceptance. Attempts to deny difference can unwittingly escalate problems as they imply that the changes are too dangerous to address. Too great an emphasis on difference can lead to unhelpful polarization and isolation. There may even be resentment about the burden of care, or disagreements about finances – whether to spend all their money on that 'once in a life-time' trip while the ill member can travel or consolidate finances to secure surviving members' future (Altschuler 1997). Differences can also contribute to problems in communication, to the extent that essential tasks such as ascertaining the ill person's wishes about future care, are neglected until too late.

The role changes required may also open new patterns of relating. In families with strong gender-defined roles, illness in a partner can mean women assume greater responsibility for executive action, enabling them to develop a new voice in relation to themselves and others (Altschuler 1997). Despite some changes in gendered roles, in many heterosexual couples it is the mother who plays the primary role in child care. In such cases, when she becomes ill, her partner may need to take on more of the child care to enable his partner to give priority to her own health. The experience of playing a greater role in caring for one's children can lead these fathers to re-evaluate how they see themselves and others (Dale and Altschuler 1997). Although the issues around stereotypically gendered roles might be different in families where parents have a same-sex relationship, illness in one partner may lead to a similar shift in the role and constructions of self of the other partner. Experiencing this change as a gain may feel threatening as it has resulted from a partner's illness. As such, it may help to include conversations about what has been learned over this time to enable these changes to be integrated in a way that feels more comfortable to all.

No loss is easy to understand. There is often a great deal of ambiguity, rendering it more difficult to know how to think or grieve. How families negotiate ambiguity is crucial to the way in which they engage with the transitions imposed by illness. Coining the phrase 'ambiguous loss', Boss (1999) draws on work with families facing Alzheimer's disease in outlining how a loved one may remain physically present but psychologically absent. She also outlines how the opposite may apply: sadness, fear, anxiety or even shame can mean that family members are physically present but emotionally unavailable. This may occur when an ill parent's distress about their own health renders them emotionally unavailable to their children.

In other situations, holding on to ambiguity enables family members to remain emotionally available despite their physical absence. Although parents may not be able to engage in *parenting activities*, they may be able to retain some level of *parental responsibility* (Parker 1993). This is crucial to both children and parents: if parenting has been core to one's sense of self, retaining an identity as a parent rather than as a patient can be tremendously helpful to one's emotional well-being (Altschuler and Dale 1999). Parents who are hospitalized may find a way of being 'present' during night-time rituals by singing or speaking to young children on the telephone at bedtime or ensuring a physical object represents their presence and containment. This notion of a continuing psychological presence despite physical absence underpins the 'memory box' that ill parents sometimes prepare for their children.

How do family boundaries change?

Drawing on work with a wide range of illness, including Alzheimer's disease, cancer and AIDS, Boss (1999), Rolland (1994) and Walker (1991) note a parallel ambiguity in the boundary of the family, suggesting that complications tend to occur when there is an overly rigid reliance on retaining a way of life that cannot be sustained. Families continue to depend on someone who is no longer able to influence the running of the household although that person remains physically present; rather than adjusting to new circumstances, situations remain 'frozen' as they were when that person was present and in good health.

Similarly, when a member is critically ill, the boundary between the family and outside world becomes more permeable, allowing non-family members such as doctors and nurses to enter and adopt roles previously the domain of mothers, fathers, brothers or sisters. In a sense, new systems evolve as people are forced to work together to maximize the ill person's chances of survival, including the patient, professionals and often only certain members of the family. This is often difficult for those who are not included, for example a second parent or members of the extended family who need to remain available to care for others in the family. Research with adults in end-stage renal failure shows poorer survival rates among the more organized and prosperous families with high rates of interdependence. The suggestion is that having been exposed to fewer experiences of loss, disorientation and boundary fluidity, highly organized families are less prepared for the chaotic pattern of illness. While it would be difficult to extrapolate too much from this work, it may well be that the patient is excluded and given up to the treatment team to enable to rest of the family to survive and retain control (Reiss *et al.* 1990).

When children are seriously ill, parents face complex boundary redefinition: they have to accept that others are more able to care for their children than themselves. They and medical professionals have to establish trust in each other while coping with whatever perceptions they have about the limitation of care provided by the other. This may present a more demanding adjustment for mothers since, despite shifts in gendered attitudes, women often remain primarily responsible for the emotional care of families.

In cases of childhood illness, additional ambiguity may develop in the boundary with educational systems. When an ill child returns to school, a teacher's role shifts from educator to emotional carer: teachers are often party to intimate information about the child and family, and are placed in a position of helping the child renegotiate their relationship with peers. Similarly, when a parent is unwell, teachers find themselves 'in loco parentis', standing in for a parent who may be temporarily or permanently unavailable to their child. In such cases, teachers may struggle to know what level of input to provide: while helping a child study or talk may enable the child to deal with what they face, stepping in too far may minimize the role of a parent who is already struggling to hold on to their identity as a parent (Altschuler *et al.* 1999).

Inevitably, the interplay between the family and professional system becomes particularly complex at times of heightened emotion. Working with illness can evoke powerful feelings of vulnerability in us all, influencing our professional and personal lives. As Sontag (1991) suggests: we all carry dual passports: one to what she calls the 'world of the healthy' and one to the 'world of the sick'. Training still tends to encourage us to distance ourselves from the impact of the work, even though the cost of trying to 'cut off' increases rather than reduces levels of stress.

We may also find ourselves acting in ways that reflect not only our own experiences but also that of the family, as we identify with and 'mirror' different aspects of family relationships. For example, relationships between team members can become strained and overly businesslike subsequent to a failed kidney transplant, as the members act out the despair and disappointment of both family and professionals. All disagreement between staff members do not reflect mirrored conflict. However, acknowledging the anger and resolving conflicts within professional teams presents families with a model that includes the idea that difficult issues can be addressed and resolved. To avoid de-skilling families and to ensure that family–professional systems function effectively, we need to move between these positions: to reflect on what illness and loss mean for ourselves as well as for the families who privilege us with their trust.

How are challenges specific to each illness?

Knowing a diagnosis provides only limited information on what illness means to any of us, so it is important to establish the nature of the condition's onset, its course, prognosis, and the incapacitation it causes (Rolland 1994). For example, the onset of a condition may be gradual, as in the usual presentation of multiple sclerosis, or acute, as with sudden heart failure. Although readjustment, problem-solving and emotional demands have some similarity in both cases, acute conditions require a more rapid mobilization of family resources and intense involvement with professionals. This influences how family members view themselves and how much illness and disability organize relationships with one another.

With some conditions, such as a stroke, there may be an initial crisis, requiring enormous adjustment in roles, after which the condition tends to stabilize. Alternatively, where a condition follows a progressive course, families experience little relief in demand and are required to adapt and change repeatedly. Where the illness is episodic or relapsing, periods of good health enable some family activities and rituals to be maintained, but the fear of recurrence may overshadow moments of health. As such, transitions between crisis and non-crisis require a readiness to negotiate often uncomfortable changes in role.

So, too, the level of incapacitation and symptom visibility affects how much people are faced with loss of identity, intimate relationship and bodily function. With conditions such as motor neurone disease, where in advanced stages one may remain cognitively intact but so physically incapacitated that it is hard to communicate, people may struggle to know whether to separate, grieve or to help the diagnosed person retain their position.

Obviously, the prognosis of a condition influences the demands families face, how each person plans for the future or values life in the presence of death. However, what we find most painful is unique to each of us: a mother with multiple sclerosis found it more difficult to bear her daughter's embarrassment at her clumsiness than what her altered gait meant for herself. Family experiences and socio-cultural beliefs affect how we understand what we are told, and how much we allow our fears to envelop our lives. Fears of death may take over as much when chances of survival are high – as with asthma – as when survival rates are poor – as with certain cancers. Some respond with seeking as much intimacy as possible, whereas others try to protect one another from the pain of parting, with distancing or exclusion.

Our past can never be separated from the present and future: how we deal with change is intricately connected with past patterns of relating and past patterns of support and disappointment. In other cases, families need the opportunity to reflect on and reconstruct aspects of their past in order to be available to one another. In other cases, the difficulties of the past have been so traumatic that the forced intimacy evoked by caring and being cared for may trigger feelings relating to prior traumatic experiences. Alongside the illness, they may find themselves experiencing flashbacks to events long forgotten. As a health professional, we may need to hold at least two dimensions in mind: the impact that illness has had on the family, and unresolved issues that pre-date the illness. In some cases, families may wish to return to issues that have burdened them for a long time. Although this may be extremely distressing, family members may feel they need to use the little time they have left to reach some resolution. In other cases, families may not wish to think about past hurt. Nonetheless, we as health professionals may need to bear in mind that such issues may exist.

How does treatment affect family life?

Treatment programmes can have a powerful regulatory and restrictive impact on relationships between family members. A proliferation in terminology for 'compliance', 'adherence', 'collaboration' and 'concordance' (Jones 2003; Sanz 2003) reflects the attempts to deal with the power imbalance and loss of control that may develop in relationships between professionals and family. Dietary restrictions, medication or procedures such as dialysis force families to rethink beliefs about personal responsibility and control: having to be watchful of a child's sugar intake inevitably affects interactions between parents and children. Families face decisions such as whether to minimize or accentuate difference, whether to ensure that everyone eats the ill person's restricted diet, and how to manage when transgressing what are usually regarded as personal boundaries, as when a mother has to adjust a catheter near the groin of the son.

The actual physiological consequences of treatment can introduce tremendous confusion: fatigue, lack of concentration or a look of depression may not indicate a change in patterns of communication or emotion. Instead, it may reflect the side-effects of medication or the fact that a drug is no longer effective and needs to be re-administered, as with medication for Parkinson's disease.

Technical advances continually alter the demands placed on families and the dynamics between family and professional systems. For example, renal failure previously meant regular haemodialysis in hospital, affecting attendance at school and work. Increased use of ambulatory dialysis at home has eased this. However, it has also meant that families have additional responsibility for performing procedures that carry a high risk of infection. Greater reliance on transplants has also presented new challenges: while employing a family donor increases the chance of a kidney or bone marrow match, success or failure carries additional meaning and may have a complex effect on subsequent family dynamics. Again, a family's experience cannot be isolated from the meaning of treatment for professionals: medical optimism about transplants has increased the frequency with which this procedure is undertaken. However, this optimism has meant that professionals have underplayed how much the affected person's life may continue to be influenced by the original disease and the drug required to avoid rejection, despite a liver or kidney transplant.

How is family life affected over time?

When someone is ill, the meaning of time may alter: the illness changes over time, just as family members move through different stages of the life cycle. Thinking first about illness, most conditions tend to follow a series of phases: initial, chronic and terminal, each presenting unique tasks. While all conditions do not follow a similar course, patient, family and professional roles shift as health alters, so that what may appear to be adaptive at one stage may not be so later.

Initially, most people experience unusual or ambiguous sensations but do not know how seriously to take this. Over time, the strength of the symptoms means that the individual and family begin to regard these symptoms as an illness. Decisions are taken about whom to tell, and attention often narrows to focus on the body, with all physical signs being scrutinized as potential indicators of disease.

Diagnosis is often the first time that professionals and family members meet, setting the terms for future collaboration. Usually, one or more family members are given information about a condition. As the shock of diagnosis can render people less able to think clearly, we now recognize the value of diagnoses being shared, of allowing time for people to absorb the news and to return to ask questions. This includes recognizing the need to help children make sense of their parents' illnesses.

In crisis phases, despite considerable panic, families and professionals tend to focus on essential assessment and life support. Whereas professionals are required to provide technical skills, to be comforting and authoritative, the tasks for the ill and healthy family members tend to be different. For example, the ill person's role may be one of providing information and following orders, learning to deal with pain, incapacitation and treatment, and forming a workable alliance with the medical team. At the same time, other family members may need to be flexible to support the treatment, while having to come to terms with their changed identity and expectations. Together or separately, they face rebuilding the meaning of their lives.

Following this, many conditions enter a chronic phase, lasting many years, and in some cases requiring ongoing vigilance, participation in complex procedures and restriction in activity. Relationships with medical professionals are often less intense now, so the boundary between family and professionals may be redrawn. Family members face such challenges as minimizing discomfort and despair, balancing caregiving with personal needs for intimacy and autonomy.

As the inevitability of death becomes apparent, caregiving tends to move from treatment towards maintaining comfort and composure. There may be a change in who is included in decisions as all prepare for the inevitability of death. As powerful feelings of grief, separation and mourning increase, many find solace in spiritual beliefs. Others may fly into action, or panic and distance themselves from the realization of the end. This may be difficult for professionals as well as families: despite the urgency to get things right, there is no best way to say goodbye, and what is most important is accepting differences in what people can tolerate.

Throughout this time, family members move through various stages in their life cycle. Transitions are characterized by upheaval and rethinking, and we all have to come to terms with our own sense of achievement and disappointment in negotiating changes in patterns of connection and separation. Although there may be considerable cultural diversity, what is probably shared is that entire three generational family systems move through periods of greater closeness and cohesion, as in early child-rearing, and periods of greater separation, as when children leave the family home. Loss of function, shifts in caretaking roles and fears of death refocus the family inwards. Where this inward focus does not coincide with the family's natural momentum, shifts in role and aspirations are particularly difficult.

Illness can impose an imbalance in the caregiving system. Two systems operate side by side: one organized around developmental issues, the other around the medical condition. While receiving care from children does not preclude caring in turn for them, extensive imbalance in generational hierarchy can limit the extent to which parents feel able to contribute to their children. At such times it can be helpful for someone outside of the family to consider what might be age-appropriate, such as schooling and contact with peers. However, here too the wider context is important: where parents are seriously ill, we as professionals need to recognize the extent to which education and friendship needs compete with the reality of a child's circumstances, that even an 8-year-old will have to assume levels of responsibility that far outweigh that of his/her peers. Even here, where possible, it helps to ensure that the levels of responsibility undertaken are manageable and do not freeze the child in a caring role they can never escape.

How does illness affect communication?

We all fluctuate in how much we wish to acknowledge what is happening to ourselves and others. So, too, we vary in what we feel we can or should share with others. Deciding what is safe to say is one of the most complex issues both families and health professionals face. In some cases it is the ill person who is readier to share what is feared, who wishes to use the little time they have left to address what is difficult.

Research indicates that where verbal and non-verbal communication matches intentions, family members' competence and physical hardiness is enhanced. The implication is that communicating openly can mitigate stressful situations (Blechman and Delamater 1993). However, it may also feel difficult to communicate openly when relating to someone who is clearly in pain or is so tired they cannot concentrate. It may feel particularly difficult to know what to say when the person with whom one wishes to speak requires onerous attention or seems to impose suffering on the lives of others. In such situations, anger, resentment and guilt may remain unacknowledged for fear of altering the fragile balance of the family.

In other contexts, it is issues related to sexuality that might be more difficult to think about. Some find that illness alters their expectations of sexual relationships, particularly where there is a paralysis, chronic pain or marked physical disfigurement. Even with psychosexual counselling aimed at exploring other ways of pleasing one another, the shock of the condition and change in appearance may leave partners reluctant to recreate or simulate the physical intimacy they once had. This is a painful decision. Silence about acknowledging grief, disappointment, revulsion, or of physically hurting one another may be aimed at protection. Far from protecting, these added boundaries widen the gap they were striving to close: just when family members most need to re-establish a shared understanding of what is happening, they may be less available to one another.

In many cases, it is the concrete aspects of a condition that are discussed openly, including dates of diagnoses, appointments, blood levels and temperatures. However, what is less frequently shared is the story of uncertainly, anxiety and fear. There may be an understandable desire to place a 'protective filter' (Judd 1989) on how much is shared with children: parents may wish to wait and assimilate news about their condition before sharing this with children. However, this does not mean these emotions do not affect interaction; rather, they influence interactions in an unvoiced and unarticulated way. Often, children know far more than adults realize. A 3-year-old who was asked why her mother was crying, answered: 'Because Mummy is sick again.' She had not been told, and in the absence of verbal input made sense of what she saw: that her mother was less attentive to her and had tears on her cheeks. Keeping frightening thoughts private over prolonged periods limits one's capacity to deal with altered living circumstances. For children in particular, such behaviour can hinder their ability to make sense of their experience, inhibiting also their ability to learn and make sense of other aspects in their lives.

Final comments: personal–professional connections

We all hold passports to the world of illness, so that the way in which we, as health professionals, interact with families is influenced by our capacity to reflect on the meaning of illness in our own lives. The work confronts us with unpredictability and ambiguity, with people who are questioning and redefining the meaning of their lives. There may be times when we question our roles, afraid of adding to their burden by conducting painful, intrusive medical procedures or talking about their illness. As such, the work can have a profound effect on us, prompting us to re-evaluate our training, expertise, and beliefs about protection, safety and childhood. Decisions about what to share undoubtedly lie with the family. Nonetheless, failing to explore certain issues unwittingly implies that those issues are too dangerous to discuss, and may reflect our own, rather than the family's, difficulty in confronting what lies ahead.

Medical diagnosis and treatment often deal in certainty – in blood counts, temperatures and blood pressure. In the face of such technology it may be difficult to value the healing power that resides in relationships in which people feel heard without having to defend themselves. Often, the best we can offer is a space in which to consider the impact of the illness and treatment on the dignity and quality of families' lives, so people can reach informed decisions that they feel comfortable with, be they about treatment, parenting or child care.

Note

This chapter draws on Altschuler, J. (1997) *Working with Chronic Illness: A Family Approach* and is published with the agreement of Macmillan Palgrave Press, UK.

References

Altschuler, J. (1997) *Working with Chronic Illness: A Family Approach*. Basingstoke: Palgrave.

Altschuler, J. (2002) Narratives of migration in therapy, *The Psychologist*, 17: 12–16.

Altschuler, J. and Dale, B. (1999) On being an ill parent, *Journal of Clinical Child Psychology and Psychiatry*, 4: 23–37.

Altschuler, J., Dale, B. and Sass-Booth, A. (1999) Supporting children when a parent is physically ill: implications for schools, *Educational Psychology in Practice*, 15(1): 25–32.

Ayalon, O. (1998) Community healing for children traumatized by war, *International Review of Psychiatry*, 10: 224–33.

Blechman, A.E. and Delamater, A.M. (1993) Family communication and Type I diabetes: a window on the social environment of chronically ill children, in R.E. Cole and D. Reiss (eds) *How Do Families Cope with Chronic Illness?* London: Lawrence Erlbaum Associates.

Boss, P. (1999) *Ambiguous Loss*. London: Harvard University Press.

Dale, B. and Altschuler, J. (1997) Different gender – different language: narratives of inclusion and exclusion, in R.K. Papadopoulos and J. Byng-Hall (eds) *Multiple Voices*. London: Duckworth.

Dwivedi, K. (1999) Sowing the seeds of cultural competence, *Context*, Special Issue, 44.

Garmezy, N. and Masten, A.S. (1994) Chronic adversities, in M. Rutter, E. Taylor and L. Hersov (eds) *Child and Adolescent Psychiatry*. Oxford: Blackwell.

Jenkins, J.M. and Smith, M.A. (1990) Factors protecting children living in disharmonious families: maternal reports, *Journal of American Academy of Child and Adolescent Psychiatry*, 29: 60–9.

Jones, G. (2003) Prescribing and taking medicines, *British Medical Journal*, 327: 819.

Judd, D. (1989) *Give Sorrow Words*. London: Free Association Press.

Kanuik, J. (1997) The Coram HIV Project: lessons from the first three years. Paper presented at the Conference on the Permanent Placement for African Children Affected by HIV/AIDS, Thomas Coram Institute, London.

Kelleher, D. and Hillier, S. (1996) *Researching Cultural Differences in Health*. London: Routledge.

Krause, I.B. (1998) *Therapy Across Culture*. London, Sage.

Krause, I.B., Rosser, R., Khiani, M.L. and Lotay, N.S. (1990) Morbidity among Punjabi medical patients in England measured by GHQ, *Psychological Medicine*, 20: 711–19.

Miah, J. (2004) Developing an integrated service of families living with HIV, *Clinical Psychology Forum*, Special Issue, *Working with Physical Illness*, 35: 25–8.

Parker, G. (1993) *With This Body*. Milton Keynes: Open University Press.

Radley, A. (1994) *Making Sense of Illness*. London, Routledge.

Reiss, D., Gonzalez, S. and Kramer, N. (1990) On the weakness of strong bonds, *Archives of General Psychiatry*, 43: 795–804.

Rolland, J.S. (1994) *Families, Illness and Disability*. New York: Basic Books.

Rutter, M. (1999) Resilience concepts and findings: implications for family therapy, *Journal of Family Therapy*, 21(2): 119–44.

Sanz, E.J. (2003) Concordance and children's use of medicines, *British Medical Journal*, 327: 858–60.

Sontag, S. (1991) *Illness as Metaphor and AIDS and its Metaphors*. Harmondsworth: Penguin.

Walker, G. (1991) *In the Midst of Winter*. London: W.W. Norton.

The prospect of death can be a time when people look for meaning in their lives. In my own practice, the development of a structured Life Review (Lester 1995) enables the dying person to talk openly about sensitive issues that are causing emotional distress. These may be feelings associated with guilt, anger, troubled family relationships, regrets and/or what they wish to accomplish before they die. This method of open communication between worker and client allows the worker to gain insight into the uniqueness of the person's life. It indicates a positive rather than negative experience for the person taking part in the process of recalling the past, the feelings associated with recording life experiences and the links with their adaptation to their current situation.

The chapter includes narrative case studies using a Life Review questionnaire to highlight a decrease in emotional pain and improved life satisfaction for the person facing death.

Background to Life Review

The theoretical foundation of Life Review was conceptualized by Butler as a normative developmental process usually associated with adults in later life. However, he did acknowledge that it could occur in younger persons who expect to die. 'The relation of the Life Review process to thoughts of death is reflected in the fact that it occurs not only in the elderly but also in younger persons who expect death, for example, the fatally ill or the condemned' (Butler 1963: 67).

Butler describes the process as a person reflecting on the course of life events in order to integrate, interpret and reorganize unresolved issues or conflicts. He also suggested that Life Review might lead to personality growth.

> As the past marches in review, it is surveyed, observed and reflected upon the ego. Reconsideration of previous experiences and their meanings occurs often with concomitant, revised or expanded understanding. Such reorganisation of past experience may provide a more valid picture giving new and significant meanings to one's life; it may also prepare one for death, mitigating one's fears.
>
> (Butler 1963: 68)

Butler's work has generated much interest, with a number of studies documenting the effects of the Life Review process on morale, life satisfaction (Haight and Bahr 1984), self-esteem (Lappe 1987) and psychological functioning in later adulthood. Research findings have emphasized the potential value of reminiscence in adjustment and adaptation in later life (Coleman 1986). Most of the literature examining any therapeutic benefits of Life Review for the terminally ill indicates the benefits of Life Review in alleviating some of the emotional distress, enabling a person to identify significant events in their life and reaffirming a sense of identity and increasing self-worth (Borden 1989; Pickrel 1989; Wholihan 1992). Self-understanding appears to enable the person to adapt to their current situation: in this instance, to prepare for death.

The basis for a structured Life Review stems from an understanding of lifespan psychology, which indicates the importance of personal growth and gives particular attention to conflict resolution and the continuing development of a person's coping strategies when facing life crises. Erikson's model of life stages and ego-integrity (1963) describes reaching integrity as the last stage of life but he did not state when this should happen – whether it be middle age or an ongoing process with a constant reaffirming of integrity at each life stage. For the person in mid-life who has never reorganized or reintegrated his accumulated experiences at each stage, facing death would mean dying with an incomplete life cycle. Using Erikson's developmental stages offers a structure for conflict resolution by review of earlier life experiences: in order to go forward, sometimes it is necessary to go backwards. However, if Erikson's integrity model can be achieved, a person could die with equanimity instead of despair, feeling a sense of wholeness.

Levinson's (1980) concept of life structure in studies of adult development provides a useful framework for understanding the developmental factors which influence the experience of life-threatening illness in younger adults. The individual life structure may be understood as the pattern of a person's life as it is seen in relationship to other persons, groups, institutions or activities. The life structure would be the border between personality and social structure, reconciling the relationship between person and environment. Levinson described it as the 'story of self in world', a concept which provides an organizing framework for the interpretation of life – a biography. He theorized that life structures emerge in early adulthood as the person separates from the family of origin, forms relationships, follows an occupational direction and forms a lifestyle based on interests, values and goals. He saw young adulthood as a time when there is a sense of fulfilment in relationships, family life and occupational advancement, but this period is also accompanied by the stress of making important life decisions. During transitional and structure-changing periods, the person reviews the past, evaluates the present life structure and considers options for change in the future, in view of new hopes and goals. Levinson described life structure changing as most pronounced during the time of mid-life transition.

The onset of a life-threatening illness means that the sense of control over the life structure, whether one is reviewing or revising existing structures, can create crisis, conflict and discontinuity. Thus, the younger terminally ill person is caught between the needs of the 'developing self', of adulthood, and the task of 'reflective self' that is generally in preparation for death in later life.

Borden (1989), in his work with young AIDS patients, suggests that the person facing a life-threatening illness tries to integrate past events with present realities in order to maintain a sense of control. He felt that Life Review might offer a therapeutic intervention to facilitate this developmental transition.

Birren and Deutchman (1991) view dying as a time to integrate and make sense of one's life as it has been lived in relation to how it might have been lived, and this is important to the adult. They described older adults as having a need to reconcile past values and goals in terms of their present realities, but acknowledge that these tasks are also needed during other life transitions, such as leaving school, job changes, entering into retirement, and so on. Birren describes Life Review as 'strengthening the fabric of life', giving the person a renewed confidence in their ability to adapt to their situation.

> You'll know better where you're going
> Because you'll know where you have been.
>   (Birren and Deutchman 1991: 7)

The psychosocial developmental theories emphasize how more meaningful transitions occurred not only in later life but also near the end of life, when future opportunities were limited. This provides an eclectic underpinning when considering Life Review work with the dying of any age.

The method

In order to formulate a questionnaire to use with the dying, I adapted Haight's schedule of the Life Review and Experiencing Form, a well-researched intervention developed in the 1980s which was used with the elderly. The resultant questionnaire is reproduced as Appendix 1 to this chapter.

The structured Life Review recognizes the importance of themes, which were developed by social scientists with background interests in the auto-biographical process. The themes recognized as the most important in people's lives are described as:

- the family
- one's career, lifework (or both)
- health and body image
- the role of money
- love and hate
- sexual identity
- experience of loss, including death
- goals and achievements
- the basis of the individual's meaning of life, set by values and beliefs

It is felt that these are powerful issues throughout a person's life and that if a person is guided through the transitional stages of the developing self (Levinson 1980), they can be helped to overcome crises.

The structured Life Review encourages the exploration of a person's life by means of sensitizing questions, covering the main themes of a person's life, provided in a one-to-one relationship built on confidentiality and trust. The Review enables the person to think about significant life events and allows them to indicate happiness, sadness, fear, achievement and regret.

The questionnaire (Appendix 1) is given to the person one week prior to commencing the work and comprises three sessions:

- Childhood/family life
- Adulthood/work life
- Here and now

Consideration is also given to the uncertainty and unpredictability of a life-threatening illness such as cancer in which the person's health can deteriorate rapidly. Also, the lack of physical and emotional energy means they may only be able to manage short periods of concentration. Therefore, it is important to offer a 'manageable task' and to finish each session on a positive aspect in case the person is not well enough to continue.

Using the structured framework, the worker's aim is to help the person recall, interpret and review past experiences within the narrative context of the Life Review process thereby developing a sense of continuity and integrity in order to prepare and face death.

Harry's story – a case study

Harry emigrated to Kenya from the UK in the 1950s; he married two years later and had two children. Africa offered a comfortable way of life until Harry sustained severe head injuries as a result of an assault. His lifestyle changed dramatically and he was forced to return to England for specialist care. He underwent a two-year rehabilitation programme when he had to learn to walk again. During the first few months of returning to England, his wife petitioned for a divorce. Harry was left with a disability, unable to walk unaided, without a home, financially insecure, without a partner and far from the country he had adopted some 30 years earlier. He managed to settle in a single-person's dwelling supported by community resources and regular contact from his grown-up children.

Harry collapsed one day and was admitted to hospital and diagnosed as suffering from terminal cancer. He was transferred to St Raphael's Hospice for an assessment of his palliative care needs. Harry presented as a frightened, anxious, lonely man who would burst into tears whenever he recalled the past few traumatic years of his life during which he had suffered multiple losses. In order to help Harry regain a sense of control and perhaps an understanding of his emotional pain, he was offered Life Review. He agreed to this and worked enthusiastically.

Summarizing the main areas of psychosocial difficulties these were: anxiety, feeling out of control, lonely, frightened, self-doubt, low self-esteem, separated from country of residence, separated from family, recently divorced and feeling life had been worthless.

The positive outcomes of Life Review

The opportunity to make sense of one's life and how it has been lived is essential for the person facing death. In the first instance, the significance for Harry in regaining personal power gave him back the control he appeared to have lost. Harry's recall of positive and negative aspects to his life helped him to identify how certain determinants had influenced his life – his 'orderly' childhood that motivated him to travel and seek adventure. He talked at length about his relationship and how selfish he had been, and admitted the marriage had been unhappy for some years. However, the most positive aspect was his two children.

Harry was able to identify past coping strategies to meet current needs and problems by evaluating his earlier coping strategies and adjustment to his disability. He was able to rekindle more passive hobbies such as reading, computers and taking an interest in natural history – these were the interests, which gave him satisfaction during his period of rehabilitation. There was clear evidence of decreased feelings of despair and improved self-esteem as Harry began to recognize a sense of continuity in his life. He was delighted that his relationship had improved with his son, who stayed with him during the final weeks of his life; this encouraged him to re-establish contact with his only brother.

Harry worked hard to reconcile past values and goals with present realities, within the limited period of time he had left. His recall of childhood experiences enabled him to recognize his spiritual needs. He had always planned to have a butterfly farm when he retired; he was content to share his existing knowledge and visit a butterfly farm in England before he died. The worker recalls how poignant this visit was for Harry (and the worker), and how his expertise in the subject enabled him to talk knowledgeably with the staff that ran the farm. At one point he was covered in butterflies – he cried with joy.

Harry had always been concerned about the amount of cognitive damage he may have sustained from his earlier assault, and because he had regained his confidence applied to MENSA and was accepted as a member before he died.

For Harry, the most precious experience of the Life Review process was the wish to improve his relationship with his children. Harry shared family stories with them which gave a greater understanding of particular periods and events which, seen from a different perspective, helped the family grow together in a time of adversity.

In the final session with Harry, he clearly was not the dying patient out of control but a person who had authority over his life and death. He described having a strong feeling that he would still belong to others after his death, by his contribution to life. He apologized to the worker for feeling 'smugly content': before Life Review Harry had said 'life had been worthless'.

For Harry, Life Review was a dynamic process. His past achievements and failures were assessed in terms of their contribution to a satisfying life structure; an acceptance of life as it had been.

Sarah's story – a user's perspective

Sarah, aged 50, was admitted to the Hospice in the later stages of her terminal illness. The nature of her cancer prevented her from leaving her bed. She presented as a quiet lady who appeared to have withdrawn from life and who communicated very little with the ward staff. She had at times suffered from periods of depression. Sarah was encouraged to talk with the social worker, and during the initial contact, when asked to describe herself, she replied: 'I am a small child with my nose pressed against the window; it is raining outside. My father is typing in the background and my brother has just died – I have been stuck as this small child all my life.'

The following, in Sarah's own written words, are extracts from her description of the experience of the Life Review process she referred to as 'journalling'. After the initial three sessions, she completed five notebooks before she died.

Doing this journalling exercise has helped me understand how the way I have 'filed' away my memories in the past, especially in my early childhood, has had a profound effect on my life. It seems as if emotions connected to sad, bad or tragic incidents have been filed with great prominence at the forefront of my 'files'. Conversely, happy, fun or pleasurable happenings and their connected emotions have been allowed to fade back into the distant part of the 'file'.

I had found, from previous attempts at self-esteem building, that writing about an event has a much more powerful effect than just thinking it through or talking it over with someone. What I had not realized was that this works just as powerfully for good and positive happenings as for bad.

If you persevere, you can reach a point where the written words help you to re-live the emotions. You can write about the incident over and over until the words just exactly describe how something feels (good or bad). This gives a great deal of relief and pleasure. Someone else reading what you have written will be able to understand how you felt at the time, or at least more nearly, and so be able to be more sympathetic and compassionate if they wish to.

It also has the effect of bringing the positive memories forward into their rightful place alongside other sadder memories. Writing about a happy memory to this depth has the effect of 'polishing up' the memory until it can shine brightly, now that it is in its proper position.

Writing about good memories has bought them into their proper position and 'shined' them up so that they have their proper, warm glowing effect in the background of my memory. Similarly with the bad things. They've been toned down and taken their proper places alongside the good rather than superseding them.

So now, I have a more balanced view of myself, my life so far now having a much less negative effect on my current emotions. It has also made it easier to understand and forgive the other people involved in the sadder memories. I also have more balanced relationships with several people, especially some in my family.

I would recommend the journalling process thoroughly. It is quite hard going to start with but becomes a real pleasure to do, and has very real effects on the poor little inner person trying to make sense of the world.

The positive outcomes of Life Review

To work with Sarah using the technique of Life Review was a most humbling experience and the worker must leave the perception of this experience to Sarah's own words.

She was observed to 'metamorphose' into a 'butterfly' during the process of Life Review work. From being a pale, weary and quiet lady, she found the emotional and physical energy to change her room – make her mark – 'dare' to do the things she had never dared do before – wear lavender, purple, hang posters on the walls, to regain her identity from youth and be happy for the first time in her life. She understood and made sense of how her life experiences had influenced her development – she worked at regaining an understanding of how earlier life determinants had moulded her life.

She was aware of the sadness and traumas she had suffered but survived, and recognized for the first time her achievements, for example she gained academic success to become a competent pharmacist. She was able to focus on her achievements even in the face of adversity and she was able to re-evaluate her entire life. Before she died, Sarah described a feeling of inner peace, enjoying her interaction with the staff and treasuring visits from her mother and sister.

The following are examples of how Life Review has been interpreted, developed and produced into a complete piece of work by the clients and how this has impacted on family members after the death of their loved one.

Fred

Fred, a 90-year-old man who was deeply troubled and overwhelmed by feelings of guilt about how contemptuously he had treated his sisters and mother when he was a young boy and in later years how badly he treated his wife and daughter. After completing Life Review, he decided to write his story in the Hospice Day Care Newsletter, using a pseudonym. This process acted as a catharsis and enabled him to understand how he had harboured a resentment for the women in his life. He recognized that, following the death of his father when he was 12 years old, he was forced to leave school and find work to provide for his mother and sisters. He was able to make peace with himself, his wife and daughter before he died.

Doris

Doris chose to tell her story and leave a permanent legacy of an embroidered tablecloth, with each corner showing a particular era of her life with symbols depicting significant events, for example the name of her favourite teacher who had inspired her at primary school and the special toys her children played with while she was bringing them up. She saw this as a family heirloom that could be handed down from generation to generation to be enjoyed at special family occasions.

Ann

Ann, a woman in her late forties, was devastated at the thought of leaving her young sons when she died. During Life Review, she had talked about distressing issues from her childhood which had remained unresolved and painful to recall. Once the process was complete, she chose to tell her story on audiotape and took the children on a journey through her childhood and work life. She described her childhood home, the fabrics of the furniture and the colours and smells. She wanted her children to remember her as they were growing up and this would be the permanent record of her existence. She would, hopefully, be a 'real' person for them to remember. Subsequently her husband used part of the tapes as a celebration of her life at her funeral.

David

David initially believed he had achieved very little in life, but during the Life Review process it transpired that, although he had started his work life as a delivery boy, he had worked his way up to become a director of the company. After David's death his daughter continued to add to his life story book by requesting that friends add their stories and memories of her father. She found this to be a great comfort during her bereavement; at her lowest ebb, she would read his story and it gave her a sense of continuity of life even in death.

Maria

Maria recalled, during the Life Review process, painful memories from the Second World War, including the loss of family members. She told the story of crossing the Austrian border on a bicycle to take food to her cousins in Germany, frequently risking being shot by border guards. Recalling these life events of which she had never spoken before, helped her to make the connection with her distress now that she was facing her own death. She was able to use humour to set free the pain and described how she had stuffed hams and sausages in her bra to take food across the border. She could not understand how the border guards could have missed the fact that when first crossing she had large breasts and on her return she had nothing.

Conclusion

The practice of social work is well used to the task of eliciting details of a client's social history, usually starting with the current situation, the presenting problem. During the course of an interview details will emerge, and the social worker focuses on those parts that they feel may have a bearing on the current situation. Nevertheless, at the end of the interview, life history may still be incomplete. A structured Life Review is an end in itself, a complete piece of work that does not replace other social work techniques and which can be used alongside methods that are more traditional. For the patients referred to in this chapter, the use of Life Review indicated improved emotional well-being and a favourable impact on family relationships after the death of the patient.

Life Review can be helpful in offering a structured way of working to clients who feel out of control of their situation and who are unable to adapt to increasing change, or are perhaps distressed by previous life events such as divorce, difficult family relationships, previous losses and disappointments.

Everyone has a story to tell, and everyone is unique. Life Review is suitable for clients who are prepared to, and want to, tell their story. Clients who are creative may wish to record their contribution in the form of poetry, paintings, scrapbooks, diaries, needlework or tapes. They need to be able to express themselves with adequate verbal or writing skills, have the mental ability to recall earlier life events and to be able to use some insight. Those suffering from cognitive impairment or severe memory loss may be therefore unable to connect past to present. It is important that the client can identify the work as treatment-focused with a serious and identified purpose. As Sheldon (1997: 68) states: 'The formal structure seems to contribute a particular sense of seriousness which adds weight to the process. It also emphasizes that the dying person is in charge since they choose the areas to review.'

Since the development of the structured Life Review questionnaire, its presentation at the Fourth Congress of the European Association for Palliative Care in Barcelona in 1995, and subsequent Life Review workshops in the UK and Europe, there has been growing evidence of its use as an effective, formal intervention, which has an evaluative component. It has been reported by professionals working within the field of palliative care (Allen, Kerr, Thompson: personal communications) that the use of the structured Life Review is a powerful vehicle for expression, allowing the person to focus outside their current situation. It can also unlock and set free what is within the person, thus acting as a catharsis for painful life experiences. It can provide the opportunity to complete an incomplete life history, which may give a more rounded view of the person. It also appears that, once the person begins their Life Review, there is renewed energy both physically and emotionally to complete the task even though life expectancy may be limited.

Bringing oneself, as a professional, into a relationship at the end of a person's life can be a daunting prospect. Life Review can provide the worker with a stimulating challenge and an opportunity to work creatively, allowing the client to achieve a sense of meaningfulness within the context of their dying. This reaffirms the original concept of Life Review and the importance of the integration of life experience and the achievement of resolution before a person dies.

The continued use of a structured Life Review will legitimize the process as a therapeutic intervention. The danger of an unstructured, non-evaluative approach could mean that Life Review may be seen as another diversional activity and in turn becoming disempowering.

Life Review clearly offers empowerment to the client, providing a unique insight into the psychological world of the dying, and therefore can be helpful with assessment procedure and care plans. Further case studies addressing the subjective experiences of the terminally ill using a structured Life Review could add to the understanding and management of the emotional and social needs of the dying.

References

Birren, J.E. and Deutchman, D.E. (1991) Guiding Autobiography Groups for Older Adults: Exploring the Fabric of Life. Baltimore: Johns Hopkins University Press.

Borden, W. (1989) Life review as a therapeutic frame in the treatment of young adults with AIDS, Health and Social Work, 14(4): 253–9.

Butler, R.N. (1963) The Life Review: an interpretation of reminiscence in the aged, Psychiatry, 26: 65–73.

Coleman, P.G. (1986) *Ageing and Reminiscence Processes: Social and Clinical Implications*. Chichester: John Wiley.

Erikson, E.H. (1963) *Childhood and Society*. New York: W.W. Norton.

Haight, B.K. and Bahr, R.T. (1984) The therapeutic role of the Life Review in the elderly, *Academic Psychology Bulletin*, 6(3): 289–99.

Lappe, J.M. (1987) Reminiscing: the Life Review therapy, *Journal of Gerontological Nursing*, 13(4): 12–16.

Lester, J. (1995) Life Review with the terminally ill. MSc dissertation, University of Southampton, UK.

Levinson, D.J. (1980) Towards a conception of the adult life course, in N.J. Smelser and E.H. Erikson (eds) *Themes of Work and Love in Adulthood*. pp. 265–90. Boston: Harvard University Press.

Pickrel, J. (1989) 'Tell me your story': using Life Review in counselling the terminally ill, *Death Studies*, 13: 127–35.

Sheldon, F. (1997) *Psychosocial Palliative Care: Good Practice in the Care of the Dying and Bereaved*. Cheltenham: Stanley Thornes.

Wholihan, D. (1992) The value of reminiscence in hospice care, *American Journal of Hospice and Palliative Care*, March/April.

Further reading

Birren, J.E. (1987) The best of all stories, *Psychology Today*, 21(5): 91–2.

Bornat, J. (ed.) (1993) *Reminiscence Reviewed: Perspectives, Evaluations, Achievements*. Milton Keynes: Open University Press.

Domino, G. and Affonso, D.D. (1990) A personality measure of Erikson's life stages: The Inventory of Psychosocial Balance, *Journal of Personality Assessment*, 54(3/4): 576–88.

Feil, N. (1985) Resolution: the final life task, *Journal of Humanistic Psychology*, 25: 91–105.

Haight, B., Coleman, P. and Lord, K. (1995) The linchpins of a successful Life Review: structure, evaluation and individuality, in B. Haight and J. Webster (eds) *The Art and Science of Reminiscing: Theory, Research, Methods and Application*. Washington, DC: Taylor & Francis.

Levinson, D.J., Darrow, C.N., Klein, E.B. *et al.* (1978) *The Seasons of a Man's Life*. New York: Alfred A. Knopf.

Lichter, I., Mooney, J. and Boyd, M. (1993) Biography as therapy, *Palliative Medicine*, 7: 133–7.

Neimeyer, G. and Rareshide, M. (1991) Personal memories and personal identity: the impact of ego-identity development on autobiographical memory recall, *Journal of Personality and Social Psychology*, 60(4): 562–9.

Nicholl, G. (1984) The Life Review in five short stories about characters facing death, *Omega Journal of Death and Dying*, 15(1): 85–96.

Rybarczyk, B. (1995) Using reminiscence interviews for stress management in the medical setting, in B. Haight and J. Webster (eds) *The Art and Science of Reminiscing: Theory, Research, Methods and Application*. Washington, DC: Taylor & Francis.

Appendix 1: Life Review questionnaire

1   CHILDHOOD / FAMILY LIFE

What is the earliest memory you have of your childhood?
What was family life like?
Would you describe yourself as a close family?
Who were you closest to in your family?
How were you punished as a child?
What was important to you as a child?
Did you feel cared for?
What were your parents' expectations of you as a child?
Was there ever illness in the family?
Do you remember being sick as a child?
Were you ever separated from someone special?
Did someone close to you die when you were growing up?
Were there other significant losses?
What did you fear most as a child?
Tell me about something you accomplished at school?
Do you remember having a best friend and sharing good times together?
Did you belong to any clubs, groups, scouts etc.?
Tell me about a happy memory from childhood – a place you liked best and why.
Would you say you enjoyed your childhood?

2   ADULTHOOD / WORK LIFE

Tell me about an important event that has happened to you in adulthood.
Tell me about your work and what it has meant to you.
Tell me of something you accomplished at work.
Did you feel appreciated in your work?
What hobbies/leisure activities were you interested in outside work?
Have you established important relationships with others?
Has religion been an important part of your adult life?
Did you marry or have a partner?
(yes)   What kind of person is/was your partner?
        Was the intimate side of your relationship important to you?
        What were your expectations of marriage? Were they fulfilled?
        Overall, would you say you had / have had a happy partnership?
(no)   Can you say why you did not marry or have a partner?
What significant losses have you experienced during your adult life?
What were they and when did they happen?
What accomplishments are you most proud of either in your family life, work life, or both?

3   HERE AND NOW

What milestones in your life do you feel have been the most major?
Why were they significant?

What would you have done differently?
How would you have changed things?
What was the happiest period in your life so far?
What made it the happiest?
What have your main satisfactions in life been?
Overall, what kind of life do you think you have had?
How do you feel you have coped with previous losses and changes?
What do you feel helped you to cope?
Have previous ways of coping helped you in your current situation?
What are the most important things in your life now?
How are you coming to terms with your illness and facing the future?
What would you like to achieve before you die?

Source: Lester 1995; adapted from Haight's Life Review and Experience Form.

6 | The death of a child

Jan McLaren

No family in western society today expects to bury a child. Yet, in 2001, in England and Wales alone, 4413 children and young people between the ages of 1 and 25 years died. A further 1103 infants died between 28 days after birth and their first birthday; 2137 babies died between birth and 27 days old; 3159 infants were stillborn; 176,364 pregnancies were terminated, and an estimated one-fifth of all conceptions resulted in spontaneous miscarriage. At every age, proportionally more boys than girls died. The causes of death were diverse and complex. Spontaneous deaths during pregnancy were related either to the health of the mother, or to the development and condition of the baby. During the first year of life, most deaths were caused by a variety of conditions originating before, during or immediately after birth. From 1 year of age up to 25, the most common cause (44 per cent) was injuries inflicted by external means, predominantly accidents; the second (13 per cent) was all forms of malignancy; the third (9 per cent) was diseases of the nervous system. The majority of deaths between age 1 and 25 years occurred suddenly, and were therefore unanticipated (Office for National Statistics 2003).

This chapter focuses on the effects upon parents of the death of a child, from age 1 to 25 years. Pregnancy and neonatal deaths are excluded as their impact is different in significant ways from that following the death of an older child. Issues facing bereaved parents are considered; similarities between them described; differences discussed; interventions which may help are identified.

In the past twenty-five years an extensive body of literature has been published, describing and analysing the impact of the death of a child upon parents. Authors include bereaved parents recounting their experience, and academics, from a range of disciplines, reporting research findings, with some drawing also upon their clinical practice. My perspective is that of a person-centred counsellor and psychotherapist. It is increasingly recognized that counselling practitioners have a role to play in research based upon what we do and what we learn from our clients about the human condition (McLeod 1999). Kvale argues extensively and persuasively that the psychoanalytical interview is a valid source of knowledge production and recognizes that this may apply equally to Rogerian therapy (Kvale 1999). Silverman advocates an integration between researcher and practitioner, recognizing our shared humanity (Silverman 2000). Feltham suggests that therapists 'may not necessarily regard themselves as exclusively and narrowly clinical workers but may regard themselves as researchers into the human condition, as data gatherers with precious gleanings to pass on to social policy makers' (Feltham 1998: 1).

As a reflective practitioner with a research background, my stance echoes that of Silverman and Feltham. What follows is derived mainly from my counselling practice since the early 1990s with 210 bereaved parents (67 couples, 68 mothers, 8 fathers) and 12 siblings. I have spent over 5000 hours meeting with bereaved clients individually, in couples and in groups. When we meet, weekly, fortnightly or monthly, I try to be entirely open to their experience. I have no agenda: how we spend our time together and the issues addressed are chosen by clients. The discourse of counselling is more than catharsis (McLaren 1998). I spend between two and three hours each session listening to parents' stories; learning about their dead children – how they lived and how they died. I hear about their relationship with each other; with the dead child, before and after death; with their surviving children, and with their extended families. I accompany their quest to find meaning in the death. We confront the reality and the enormity of their loss. I facilitate their emotional expression of grief. I provide emotional and cognitive support as they struggle to find some purpose in continuing their own lives, enabling them to create a new normality in a chaotic and unrecognizable world. I strive to understand accurately what they tell me and to convey my understanding empathically, checking that I have not misunderstood. I offer my acceptance of their thoughts, feelings and behaviour, rather than reassurance or judgement. I do not hide behind a professional veneer or affect to be a blank screen upon which clients may project feelings. Rather, I reveal my authenticity as a human being, transparent in conveying my genuine interest in and concern for my clients. As an outsider I do not need to be protected from their worst thoughts and feelings. I regard myself as a companion and witness to their experience, as their grief evolves over the months, years, that I remain alongside them.

My clinical practice forms the basis of this chapter, supplemented by quotations from 50 hours of tape-recorded, semi-structured interviews with 10 per cent of former clients, undertaken, at least two years after their loss, as qualitative research into their experience. I have also, where appropriate, referred to key texts in the field of parental bereavement; these are supplemented by suggestions for further reading at the end of the chapter.

The impact of the death of a child

Conventional wisdom, across the centuries and transcending cultural boundaries, asserts that parental bereavement following the death of a child is more traumatic, protracted, profound and complex than any other bereavement (Rando 1986), and that the death of a child is the most tragic and unjust of all losses. The validity of such claims was challenged by Dijkstra and Stroebe (1998). They considered most studies of parental grief to be methodologically flawed, as they lack a carefully matched comparison population. What may be acknowledged unequivocally, however, is that for most bereaved parents the death of a child is the single worst experience of their lives. As one father told me, 'The only thing that could be worse than losing my son would be if my daughter died too.' A child's death is contrary to the biological law of the universe, which determines that the old should die before the young. When this law is broken there is a sense of outrage and disbelief. For the immediate mourners there evolves an awareness that their hopes and expectations for the future have changed irrevocably. There will always be a void in the family: the death of a child is for ever (Rubin 1993). The specific impact of a child's death will vary from person to person. No two people grieve in the same way, at the same pace, or over the same period of time. The emotional and cognitive processes of adjusting to the loss are rarely synchronized between parents: commonly, misunderstandings arise and a breakdown in communication occurs. In summary, 'the death of a child may thus precipitate an existential crisis wherein the basic security and meaning of life and interpersonal relationships are brought violently into question' (Oliver 1999: 199).

Factors affecting parental bereavement

There are many factors which contribute to individual differences between parents following the death of a child: these include the nature, meaning and quality of the lost relationship; the age and personality of the child at death; characteristics of the mourner such as personality, age, physical and psychological health, and previous experience of loss; the social, economic, cultural, ethnic and religious background of the parents; the nature of relationships within the immediate and extended family; the stage the immediate family is at in its life cycle; and the manner and circumstances of the death.

Gender

While there are undisputed gender-specific effects of losing a baby, thereafter the reported differences transcend gender boundaries. I have become aware of an assumption prevalent in western society, that a mother's grief is worse than that of a father (Finkbeiner 1996). As a bereaved teenage sibling expressed so poignantly, several years after his brother's death, 'People come to the house and they always ask, "How's your mum coping?" What about my dad? They never ask about him or about how I am! My dad's heart is broken but he doesn't show it as much as my mum. So, they assume he's OK. But I live with them and I know differently.'

In my clinical practice, I hesitate to focus too intently upon innate gender differences: my bereaved clients are individual people. Changes in the structure of western society have led to a crossover of roles within many families, across generations and social class. Women are employed outside the home at all stages of their children's lives, whereas increasing numbers of men share home-making, domestic duties and child care; some work from home and may regard themselves as house husbands. It would be interesting to study the impact these social changes have had upon the expression of grief in the men and women involved. Whatever the causes, it is evident that the cultural stereotypes of men being emotionally inhibited in their response to loss, and of women freely expressing their emotions, do not reflect the reality as experienced in my clinical practice.

Sudden death

The sudden death of a child results in commonly held assumptions about life being shattered. In one instant much that constitutes a normal life has changed and parents are profoundly traumatized, barely able to function. This may be their first encounter with death: they may not even be aware of the practical procedures which may follow: police interviews; media intrusion; a post mortem; the funeral; burial or cremation; a coroner's inquest; a court hearing. Parents are immersed in the immediate practicalities of disposing of the body. Invariably the funeral is over and the family left to resume a 'normal' life within two weeks.

In the early months, bereaved parents describe themselves as 'being like zombies, on automatic pilot'. They appear to be frozen emotionally, dissociated from the reality of everyday life. They go through the motions of maintaining a routine but find themselves forgetful and unable to concentrate. Many feel profoundly exhausted; they sleep and eat too much or too little; some have physical symptoms which echo those of their child at death; many describe a sense of tightening in the throat and an ache around the heart. Most do not recognize themselves and fear they are going mad.

At this time most parents are unable to engage in any close communication with others. To their partners and children they seem remote and withdrawn. Sexual intimacy between partners may feel inappropriate: even cuddling or holding may be intrusive. For some, however, close physical contact may bring comfort and ease feelings of loneliness. Love-making may be a bitter sweet reminder of the conception of their child. A father whose teenage son died in a road accident, explained,

> We actually made love within a couple of days of Ben dying. And we both wanted to. And you'd think, how on earth could you? But, the way I've worked it out in my own brain, is that we are animals and it would seem absolutely, perfectly logical if it was an animal, who'd lost its litter, to mate immediately, and try to make another litter. You wouldn't think anything of it. It's only because we're human we think, how weird, that's got to be mad. But ultimately we are animals. But I was shocked. I mean you wonder whether you are mad or not. How could you? After that there was probably a very, very long break before we made love again, but in terms of months not years.

Often, when others attempt to reach out towards them, parents have difficulty responding. They are overwhelmed by the trauma of their child's death and are absorbed in their grief. Depending upon their age, siblings may find themselves literally caring for their parents. 'They almost needed me to breathe for them,' reported a 17-year-old youth. Many parents, years later, are unable to recall much about this period. As time passes, they emerge from their frozen state to experience the emotional, cognitive and practical reality of their child's death. Everything may feel very much worse before it feels better.

Anticipated death

When a child dies following terminal or chronic illness, parents have already suffered the loss of the healthy child, or, when the condition was congenital, the loss of a normal child. Grieving precedes the death. Although the child's death was anticipated, this fact may not have been accepted. The timing and manner of death cannot always be predicted or controlled. Prior to death, family life may have centred around the sick child. Even when the terminal illness was brief, family routines have been disrupted by clinical appointments, inpatient and outpatient hospital care, the adaptation of the home to accommodate special needs, and the interruption of family activities. When the child dies, the family loses its focus. One or both parents may find themselves with time on their hands, time which was previously yearned for but which now emphasizes the void left by the child. Initially, overwhelmed by grief, they are unable to resume normal family activities. Immediately after death the family will lose social security benefits which may have been awarded to support the special needs of the child and have been relied upon to sustain the family (Corden *et al.* 2001). One or both parents may have given up paid work to look after the child but find themselves unable to gain immediate re-employment. Parents may be physically and emotionally exhausted after caring for their child. Relationships with professional staff and other families with a sick child may be severed abruptly, resulting in secondary losses associated with the extended community which knew the child. In addition to the complex thoughts and feelings associated with any death, parents may question the purpose of the suffering endured by the child. If death was inevitable, why did the child have to undergo invasive and often mutilating treatment? Relief that the suffering is over is accompanied by guilt.

Siblings may share their parents' relief that the suffering is over. Ambivalence towards the dead child is common. Sometimes they will have witnessed horrific changes in their sibling's body as a result of their illness, and they retain terrifying images of disfigurement which haunt them. They may suffer hypochondriosis and fear that they too will become ill and die. They may harbour feelings of deep resentment towards the child following the disruption of their own lives during the period of illness. They may have felt acute embarrassment in having a sibling who was conspicuously different from their peers. They think such feelings should be concealed as they believe they are expected to have only compassion for a sick child. Having sometimes wished the child dead, either because the suffering was unbearable to witness, or because they longed for a return to family normality, siblings may feel responsible for the death and be consumed by a sense of guilt. Siblings may have lost their best friend, rival, companion or mentor. They may miss the opportunities they had to love and to care for their sibling: the sick child may have become the central focus of their lives as well as the lives of their parents.

Following the death, siblings may be hopeful that their parents will now have the time, energy and desire to pay attention to their needs. If they remember a time before the child was ill, they may hope for a resumption of a more normal family life. Such hopes are rarely realized in the immediate aftermath of the death. Parents remain preoccupied with the dead child, unaware of the complex feelings and needs of their surviving children.

Death of an only child

While parents who lose an only child endure all the consequences attributed to parents who have surviving children, they have the additional trauma of losing their role, identity and status in society as parents (Talbot 1996). Younger parents may have another child but parents who are now infertile do not have that choice. The father of a teenage son, who died within a year of developing bone cancer, encapsulates the finality of the loss:

> Simon was our only child. Jane and I are both only children and from our point of view the loss of Simon was totally devastating. I suppose invariably, for whatever reason one has children, one knows they are going to outlive one, that family myths and legends and family belongings will likely be passed on. I had been very keen on family history research. The three of us had dragged around churchyards, record offices, on wet mornings, foggy days, whatever. This was Simon's heritage. But suddenly there was no point in that any more when Simon died. Then, having to make a will and sit with a lawyer and go through what we wanted to happen to our property, being the end of the dynasty, was a harsh, horrible reality, which was very difficult to do. Now there's no one to pass anything on to. History stops here for this family.

Extended families

Where parents have divorced before the child's death, new partners and half-brothers and sisters may, also, be grieving but their suffering may not be acknowledged. Sometimes ex-partners may grow closer, having discussed funeral arrangements and memorials, and shared memories of the child. This reminder of their previous relationship can be threatening to second partners but can also be an opportunity for both families to grow closer. Single parents may no longer be in contact with their previous partner and, like widows or widowers who have lost a child, may be alone in their grief. Grandparents suffer a double grief: they not only mourn their grandchild but they also grieve for the lost hopes of their own child, the bereaved parent. In supporting their children and surviving grandchildren, grandparents may find their own distress and needs unacknowledged. When grandparents are elderly or frail, and even when they are not, they may question why they should remain alive but their grandchild die; their child, the bereaved parent, may ask the same question about their parents and even sometimes about themselves.

Issues shared by bereaved parents

In considering issues which are significant for the relationship of bereaved parents, it is important firstly to identify the thoughts and feelings which they have as individuals (Gilbert 1996). When a child dies, parents lose a part of themselves which is irreplaceable: 'losing Jack was like an amputation'. No matter how many other children they have, the loss is particular to the unique and special relationship they had with this child. Mothers have carried the child within their body during pregnancy, and many fathers feel a similar bond, that their child is a part of them. 'I expected to live on in him and in his children after him.' Parents' hopes and expectations for the future may have been invested in this child. A biological and spiritual link with immortality is severed.

Fundamental to all parents is a sense of responsibility for the nurturing and protection of their young, no matter what age. When a child dies, most parents feel an acute and persistent sense of failure and guilt that they were unable to protect their child. They acknowledge this is irrational, but they have a primitive sense that they should have known their child was going to die and they should have been able to prevent it. Commonly, both parents lose self-confidence. This may be the result of their failure to protect their offspring. Equally, they may no longer trust a world where their basic assumptions about life have been shattered. If a child can die, anything can happen. Many parents live in fear for each other and, in particular, for their surviving children: 'Just because you've lost one doesn't mean you won't lose another.' Some have little fear for themselves: their own death may reunite them with the child; suicidal ideation occurs. Meanwhile, they face an indeterminate future without their child. Whenever they see children who look, move or sound like their child, or are the same age, they are reminded of them. Whenever the child's peers attain developmental landmarks, they are reminded of what should have been. A child is remembered as being eternally the age at which they died, while simultaneously parents fantasize about how the child would be at their chronological age.

For most parents, one of the primary tasks of grieving is to find an enduring place for the dead child in their lives (Klass 1997). These parents acknowledge the reality and finality of the physical death but strive to integrate the child into their ongoing lives. Some people experience a sense of the child's presence. Many dream vividly about their children: initially dreams may be nightmares about the death but, as years pass, they incorporate the child at different ages, reliving the reality of those former times. Parents with a faith in an afterlife have a strong belief that their child lives on and acknowledge an evolving relationship with the child (Klass 1999). Most continue to think and talk about their children, sharing memories of their lives, wondering what they would have done in certain circumstances, discussing what their opinions would have been, pursuing interests the children had, doing things on their behalf – living for them. Many parents conduct imaginary conversations with their children. Some parents raise funds to create memorials in their child's name or to support research into conditions which caused their death or to fund medical support for sick children, or counsellors for the bereaved. Parents' continuing bonds with their dead children take many forms.

Most bereaved siblings strive similarly to find a continuing place for their dead brother or sister in their lives. This place may evolve as the sibling grows older. No matter what the sibling's chronological age, he usually continues to think of the dead child as younger or older depending upon his order in the family. Children born after a child has died may create a relationship in fantasy with their dead sibling and may continue to draw upon this for inspiration or companionship, or as a role model or mentor, as they grow up.

Commonly, parents describe feeling physically and emotionally vulnerable during the early years of grief. A longitudinal study of 21,062 bereaved parents in Denmark concluded that the death of a child is associated with an overall increased mortality from both natural and unnatural causes in mothers. Both mothers and fathers were significantly vulnerable to death from unnatural causes in the first three years after the child's death (Li et al. 2003).

Parental grief is not static but evolves with an idiosyncratic, multifaceted and unpredictable momentum. Most parents acknowledge that the pain of the loss never goes away completely: it recurs with a familiar severity, but less frequently, and diminishes more rapidly than in earlier years. Many parents echo what this father of a teenage son stated so eloquently: 'A day doesn't go by without I think of Tim; without I remember Tim; without I miss Tim.' Parents do not 'get over the death. You simply learn to live with it.' They learn to smile and laugh again, and to take an interest in life: good memories of the child's life supersede those of the child's death. But, as one mother said: 'There's always an edge to things. Nothing will ever be the same again.'

Effects on the parents' relationship

There is unequivocal agreement that the death of a child creates a profound strain upon the parents' relationship. This does not necessarily precipitate a permanent breakdown (Oliver 1999). In a review of studies of parental relationships, Dijkstra and Stroebe (1998) found that some deteriorated, others reported no change, whereas others improved. In a review of literature concerning the incidence of divorce among bereaved parents, Schwab (1998) concluded that only a small proportion of bereaved parents divorce as a consequence of the death: there may be both positive and negative effects on the relationship. Much depends upon the quality of the relationship prior to the child's death. In my own clinical work, 3 per cent of relationships have subsequently broken up. Most couples report being close and mutually supportive immediately after the death but become less available to each other as weeks pass. They become closer again as they begin to acknowledge, understand and to respect the uniqueness of their partner's process: this may take months, even years.

What are the significant issues that affect the relationship between parents? The underlying problems arise from the differences in the ways each parent experiences the loss. Unless they have previous experience of death, most newly bereaved parents do not realize that people grieve differently. They are shocked and dismayed to find their partner thinking, feeling and behaving differently from themselves. Some people believe their partner cannot be grieving if they are not manifesting distress as they do. There can develop a hierarchy of grievers; members of a family believing they are the chief mourner or the only one to grieve. Partners may become hypersensitive to each other's moods and engage in highly protective behaviour, often when this is not wanted. They may feel they have to be 'strong' for each other, which usually involves suppressing their own thoughts and feelings. Sometimes partners become impatient with the persistence of the other's depression and absorption in the loss. They may be struggling heroically to find something positive in life and become debilitated and angered by their partner's inability or apparent refusal to do the same. These differences are so fundamental that couples feel alienated from each other and consequently they feel desperately lonely (Riches and Dawson 2000). At the time when they need each other the most, to provide solace, support, understanding and security, they simply cannot 'be there' for each other. Each is preoccupied with grief for the child. They have a secondary loss – that of each other.

When either parent has been involved in any way with the death, perhaps when the cause was an accident, not only may that parent feel responsible but the other parent may also attribute blame, whether or not this is justified. When death was the result of a medical condition, either parent may feel responsible for conveying a genetic predisposition to this, especially when there have been similar deaths in the family. To be blamed by one's partner for a child's death is a devastating insult. When one parent is actually responsible for the death, the future of the relationship is significantly jeopardized.

Most parents strive to find a meaning for the death (Braun and Berg 1994). Philosophically and spiritually they have a profound need to know why this happened. One partner may find answers through a religious faith and be sustained by this; another may reject religion altogether. Many parents echo what Ben's father explained:

If we knew Ben was in a wonderful place and he is really very happy, and it is a better place than it is here, that would be such a comfort. You could accept it all then. You could accept it all other than the fact that he's not here and you can't talk to him and you're lonely without him. Knowing, of course, as well that there's life after death, and that one day we are all going to be back together again. I could settle for that and get on with my own life.

Some parents visit spiritualists in the hope that their child will communicate through a medium. This can cause problems between parents when one is suspicious of charlatans and anxious to protect the other from emotional manipulation. One may feel envious if the child 'comes through' to their partner but not to them.

Conflict between couples may arise over practical issues such as the disposal or retention of the child's possessions. Decisions have to be made, and reviewed as time passes, over how the child's room is used; whether or not photographs of the child are displayed; how frequently the grave should be visited; what should be done with the child's ashes; how the child's birthday and the anniversary of the death are commemorated; how parents can be supportive of each other at significant times in the calendar, such as Christmas, their own birthdays and those of their surviving children. How can they cope with extended family occasions when their child is conspicuously absent? One of the most stressful events is the wedding of a surviving sibling. The dead child may have been the obvious choice for bridesmaid or best man. Who dares to fill that role? The wedding photographs become a symbol of a ruptured family rather than a memento of a new union. Observing physical and psychological characteristics in other family members, including each other, may be a painful reminder of the dead child which reinforces the sense of loss; conversely, such similarities may bring comfort.

For some parents, the family home becomes a sanctuary, the only place where they feel safe and protected from an unsafe world. For others, the home is a constant reminder of the dead child. If one parent wishes to stay at home, whereas the other prefers to go out, conflict will arise. Sometimes one parent accedes to the other's need; but when this happens the compromising partner will frequently become resentful. On other occasions parents go their separate ways, and eventually the couple may drift apart as they spend less and less time together. Similar issues arise over holidays. One parent may be fearful to go away: fearful of being surrounded by families with children, poignant reminders of happier times; fearful of meeting new people who will ask about their children; fearful of going away and leaving surviving children who may come to harm. The other parent may long to retreat from daily reminders of their loss, into a different and stimulating environment which holds no memories of their child, where they can be anonymous and are unlikely to encounter anyone who knows them and their circumstances: contrasting needs which feel irreconcilable.

As part of revising their assumptions about the world, many parents experience a radical change in values. They recognize that tomorrow may never come, and may find this liberating. Their attitude to money may become cavalier, they spend extravagantly to comfort themselves. Surviving siblings may be indulged materially, rules relaxed, boundaries extended, not always in their best interests. Some parents resign from work which they had previously merely tolerated. They retire early or seek alternative employment which is more congenial. This can be constructive but may cause problems for couples where one parent feels they are subsidizing the freedom of choice taken by the other. Many parents report a different perspective on matters which previously would have been distressing. A psychiatrist expressed puzzlement when a mother appeared to accept calmly her much loved, elderly father's diagnosis of Alzheimer's disease. 'When you've lost your son at the age of 20, everything else pales into insignificance. My father has lived his life: my son wasn't given that chance.' Although most feel empathy and compassion for other bereaved parents, many find themselves exasperated and unsympathetic towards people who have lost a pet, or a material possession, or a job and who expect them to understand 'because you have lost your child'. There is simply no comparison.

Help for bereaved parents

The needs of bereaved parents are as varied and complex as their experience of grief. In the immediate aftermath of the death, basic practical help to facilitate a daily routine is appreciated. Such support, which maintains family functioning, is usually provided by the extended family, friends, neighbours and colleagues. As time passes and parents become immersed in their grief, this support may be withdrawn: parents are unable to articulate their needs and helpers lose confidence in their ability to help. The wider community moves on, unaware of what is happening to parents who feel left behind, misunderstood and increasingly isolated.

At a time of transition from one way of life to a 'new normality', when fear, uncertainty and profound distress prevail, a counsellor may provide a secure base where bereaved parents can share their thoughts, feelings and behaviours about the past, present and future. As one of the fundamental causes of relationship disharmony is parents not understanding each other's process, meeting with a counsellor may address and alleviate this situation. A useful model in clinical practice is to have a three-session rotation: I meet separately with each parent and in the third session I meet both together. In the individual sessions the parents are able to talk about and express their thoughts and feelings, without inhibition, to an empathic and acceptant listener. Each parent approaches the joint sessions knowing that their experience has been acknowledged and understood, believing that I am concerned for both partners, that I do not take sides or believe that one is right and the other wrong. Their 'rehearsal' of significant issues with me gives them the confidence to explore these further with each other in my presence, if they wish, both trusting that I will be supportive. Communication between them is facilitated; respect and understanding of each other's perspective follows. The aim of the session is not to change each other but to accept and to accommodate their differences. They may, as part of this process, discuss strategies to employ, together or individually, to support themselves, each other and the relationship. With this pattern of therapeutic involvement continuing over time, many couples find their ability to communicate and to care for each other, both in and away from the counselling sessions, is greatly enhanced.

When couples acknowledge that their grief is different and that there is no single 'right' way to grieve, they may become more tolerant of each other and more sensitive to each other's moods and needs. When one partner is having a 'bad' day they may hesitate to communicate this for fear of spoiling a good day for their partner. The oscillation between bad and good days, loss orientation and restoration, fits readily into Stroebe and Schut's dual process model of grief (Stroebe and Schut 1999). In time, many couples learn to tell each other when they are feeling especially raw and will consult each other about what they most need to help them through a bleak period.

Groups for bereaved parents, facilitated either by a counsellor or by other parents who are further on in their grief, can be highly therapeutic. The main benefit of a group is a realization for parents that they are not alone, that others have suffered a similar fate, sometimes even worse than their own. They discover that others will identify with, will understand and will accept their thoughts, feelings and behaviour. They become aware that group members are interested to learn about their dead child and, in time, will feel they know the child. They are conscious of practical and emotional support being offered; reciprocally, they are able to use their experience and understanding to help other group members. They learn practical tips on how to respond in a diverse range of situations. Significantly, 'this is a place where we feel we can really be ourselves. We don't have to pretend or put on a front. When we meet, it doesn't matter if we're having a bad day. Others in the group will be feeling OK and they will be there for us. Another day we'll do the same for them.' But, 'of course, this is a group which no one ever wants to be eligible to join.'

Close friendships are formed in therapeutic groups, often replacing those of existing friends who were unable to sustain a continuing relationship with bereaved parents. It is difficult to be a friend to bereaved parents, especially at a time when they are emotionally labile, highly sensitive, vulnerable, prone to take offence, indecisive, and distracted by grief. Many parents recognize that their friends 'cannot win: some days we want to be asked how we are; on others we don't wish to talk about what's happened.

We can't predict how we will be from one day to the next, so it's not surprising they don't know what to do. It's usually better if we initiate contact but we don't always have the energy or the inclination.'

Younger parents may decide to have another baby. When they do, the new child can have a healing and cohesive influence, providing a new focus and purpose for the family. But the family remains incomplete: there is always one member missing.

In time, many parents take comfort in their surviving children. They enjoy their company and delight in their progress: grandchildren are a source of new life and hope. But there may be continuing reminders that they are not the child who was lost, and sometimes parents fail to appreciate the surviving children's unique qualities. Parents of older children have reported that, over the years, these young people have assumed some of the characteristics of the dead child so that they become an amalgam of themselves and their sibling. Other siblings find they need to distance themselves from parents who have become overprotective and overindulgent, and who continue simultaneously to seem overinvolved with the dead child. Many find the chasm which arose between them in the early years, is insurmountable. Siblings have found respite from the oppressive grief of their parents among their peers, following normal educational routines and socializing away from the family home. Many bereaved siblings feel they not only lost a brother or sister but their parents as well.

As surviving siblings leave home, many parents seek new activities for their nurturing and creative instincts. Domestic pets become surrogate children. Gardens are a source of satisfaction. Imaginative cooking enables parents to nurture each other. Creative arts and crafts such as painting, drawing, photography, music-making, dancing, joinery, pottery, needlecraft and writing, provide outlets for emotional expression and distraction from grief. Exercise and keeping fit provide a way to integrate mind and body. Study can extend a parent's intellectual and social environment. Whether these activities are undertaken alone or in the company of others, they all serve to help parents find a new purpose in living.

Conclusion

Although individuals grieve, they do so in the context of their families and the wider community. Each affects the other. I have focused predominantly here upon the social sub-system which is a partnership between parents. Many of the issues affecting mothers and fathers impact upon siblings and the extended family. But their experience of grief is different. Death and bereavement are featuring more prominently in the media than ten years ago: death in the western world is no longer a taboo subject. Heightened awareness and better understanding of the diverse and multidimensional consequences of death, starting in the family and extending through school, the workplace and the wider community, will help to attenuate the distress caused to bereaved people by the ignorance of others. Perhaps we should all try to acknowledge death and accept its inevitability. Then, possibly, we will be better able to support the bereaved in our communities as they undergo the turbulent process of grieving for their loved ones.

References

Braun, M.J. and Berg, D.H. (1994) Meaning reconstruction in the experience of parental bereavement, *Death Studies*, 18: 105–29.

Corden, A., Sainsbury, R. and Sloper, P. (2001) *Financial Implications of the Death of a Child*. London: Family Policy Studies Centre.

Dijkstra, I.C. and Stroebe, M.S. (1998) The impact of a child's death on parents: a myth (not yet) disproved?, *Journal of Family Studies*, 4(2): 159–85.

Feltham, C. (ed.) (1998) *Witness and Vision of the Therapists*. London: Sage.

Finkbeiner, A.K. (1996) *After the Death of a Child: Living with Loss through the Years*. Baltimore: Johns Hopkins University Press.

Gilbert, K.R. (1996) 'We've had the same loss, why don't we have the same grief?' Loss and differential grief in families, *Death Studies*, 20: 269–83.

Klass, D. (1997) The deceased child in the psychic and social worlds of bereaved parents and during the resolution of grief, *Death Studies*, 21: 147–75.

Klass, D. (1999) *The Spiritual Lives of Bereaved Parents*. Philadelphia: Brunner/ Mazel.

Kvale, S. (1999) The psychoanalytic interview as qualitative research, *Qualitative Inquiry*, 5(1): 87–114.

Li, J., Precht, D.H., Mortensen, P.B. and Olsen, J. (2003) Mortality in parents after death of a child in Denmark: a nationwide follow-up study, *The Lancet*, 361(1 February): 363–7.

McLaren, J. (1998) A new understanding of grief: a counsellor's perspective, *Mortality*, 3(3): 275–90.

McLeod, J. (1999) *Practitioner Research in Counselling*. London: Sage.

Office for National Statistics (2003) *Mortality Statistics DH3 (28)*. London: Office for National Statistics.

Oliver, L.E. (1999) Effects of a child's death on the marital relationship: a review, *Omega*, 39(3): 197–227.

Rando, T.A. (ed.) (1986) *Parental Loss of a Child*. Illinois: Research Press Company.

Riches, G. and Dawson, P. (2000) *An Intimate Loneliness: Supporting Bereaved Parents and Siblings*. Buckingham: Open University Press.

Rubin, S.S. (1993) The death of a child is forever: the life course impact of child loss, in M. Stroebe, W. Stroebe and R.O. Hansson (eds) *Handbook of Bereavement: Theory, Research and Intervention*. Cambridge: Cambridge University Press.

Schwab, R. (1998) A child's death and divorce: dispelling the myth, *Death Studies*, 22: 445–68.

Silverman, P.R. (2000) Research, clinical practice, and the human experience: putting the pieces together, *Death Studies*, 24: 469–78.

Stroebe, M. and Schut, H. (1999) The dual process model of coping with bereavement: rationale and description, *Death Studies*, 23: 197–224.

Talbot, K. (1996) Mothers now childless: survival after the death of an only child, *Omega*, 34(3): 177–89.

Further reading

De Vries, B., Dalla Lana, R. and Falck, V.T. (1994) Parental bereavement over the life course: a theoretical intersection and empirical review, *Omega*, 29(1): 47–69.

Hagemeister, A.K. and Rosenblatt, P.C. (1997) Grief and the sexual relationship of couples who have experienced a child's death, *Death Studies*, 21: 231–52.

Kirschenbaum, H. and Henderson, V. (1990) *The Carl Rogers Reader*. London: Constable.

Kissane, D.W. (2002) Shared grief: a family affair, *Grief Matters: The Australian Journal of Grief and Bereavement*. 5(1): 7–10.

Klass, D. (1988) *Parental Grief: Solace and Resolution*. New York: Springer.

Klass, D., Silverman, P.R. and Nickman, S.L. (eds) (1996) *Continuing Bonds: New Understandings of Grief*. Washington, DC: Taylor & Francis.

Klass, D. and Walter, T. (2001) Processes of grieving: how bonds are continued, in M.S. Stroebe, R.O. Hansson, W. Stroebe and H. Schut, (eds) *Handbook of Bereavement Research: Consequences, Coping and Care*. Washington, DC: American Psychological Association.

Knapp, R.J. (1986) *Beyond Endurance: When a Child Dies*. New York: Schocken.

Lehman, D.R., Lang, E.L., Wortman, C.B. and Sorenson, S.B. (1989) Long-term effects of sudden bereavement: marital and parent–child relationships and children's reactions, *Journal of Family Psychology*, 2(3): 344–67.

Mearns, D. and Thorne, B. (1999) *Person-centred Counselling in Action*. London: Sage.

Mearns, D. and Thorne, B. (2000) *Person-centred Therapy Today: New Frontiers in Theory and Practice*. London: Sage.

Nadeau, J.W. (1998) *Families Making Sense of Death: Understanding Families*. Thousand Oaks, CA: Sage.

Rosenblatt, P.C. (2000) *Parental Grief: Narratives of Loss and Relationship*. Philadelphia: Brunner/Mazel.

Sanders, C.M. (1992) *Surviving Grief and Learning to Live Again*. New York: John Wiley.

Sarnoff Schiff, H. (1977) *The Bereaved Parent*. London: Penguin.

Schwab, R. (1992) Effects of a child's death on the marital relationship: a preliminary study. *Death Studies*, 16: 141–54.

Stroebe, M.S., Hansson, R.O., Stroebe, W. and Schut, H. (2001) *Handbook of Bereavement Research: Consequences, Coping and Care*. Washington, DC: American Psychological Association.

7 | Interventions with bereaved children

Grace H. Christ

In the USA, at any given time more than 2 million children and adolescents have experienced the death of a parent. Although this represents 3.4 per cent of the population under 18 years of age, it is only during the past two decades that children's responses to a parent's death have been studied prospectively. Earlier studies relied on the reflections of adults who, as children, had lost a parent or on the findings of researchers seeking causal connections between loss in childhood and adverse mental health outcomes in adulthood. Findings from these retrospective studies often were contradictory (Crook and Eliot 1980; Van Eerdewegh et al. 1985; Tennant 1988; Saler and Skolnick 1992; Tremblay and Israel 1998); however, they strongly suggested that children's adaptation was affected more by the events surrounding the parent's death and its aftermath, by the presence of more stressors and by the balance between risk and protective factors than by the death itself. The mediators identified most consistently as affecting the course and outcome of children's bereavement are the quality of child care after the loss, the child's relationship with the surviving parent, and aspects of the child's risk and resilience (Tennant et al. 1980; Bifulco et al. 1987, 1992; Harris et al. 1987; Breir et al. 1988; Saler and Skolnick 1992; Sandler et al. 1992; Worden 1996).

The more recent growth in research on child bereavement has expanded the evidence base for interventions. Pynoos (1992) described the expansion as a result, in part, of a 'quiet revolution' that took place throughout psychiatry and other mental health disciplines as the barriers against interviewing children directly were removed, with the result that studies could include the self-reports of children as additional sources of information. Incorporating new interviewing techniques with children and developmentally sensitive instruments, these studies continue to provide important longitudinal data.

A broad range of bereavement interventions have been described in the clinical practice literature. Common approaches have included the following:

- providing anticipatory guidance with both parents and children before the death occurs during a terminal condition;
- enhancing parents' knowledge, competence and communication with their children after the death;
- helping children and parents understand, express and manage their own grief reactions;
- supporting the children's development of their own internal relationship with the lost parent as well as their relationship with the surviving parent;
- addressing practical problems and minimizing the effects of adverse secondary changes after the death: for example, sudden family moves, separation experiences or other negative events;
- facilitating the children's reintegration into school;
- helping families cope with the many changes that occur within the family after a parent dies: for example, household management, teaching, discipline and emotional nurturing;
- promoting new relationships and developing supportive networks for bereavement;
- helping children master new developmental challenges and develop a satisfying life experience without the lost parent's day-to-day presence.

In recognition of the important interaction between parent and child, interventions increasingly include work with both children and parents (Schafer 1965; Kranzler *et al.* 1990; Siegel *et al.* 1990; Worden 1996; Punamaeki *et al.* 1997; Raveis *et al.* 1999; Rotheram-Borus *et al.* 2003; Sandler *et al.* 2003a; Sandler *et al.* 2003b). Group approaches as well as individual counselling have been expanding within community agencies and schools to help bereaved children cope with a range of difficulties in maintaining schoolwork and peer relationships after a parent's death. School bereavement groups and individual counselling often include children experiencing loss resulting from a parent's death as well as loss resulting from divorce.

Sensitivity to developmental differences in children's ways of processing grief is increasingly reflected in many bereavement groups and in individual counselling. The sheer size of the parentally bereaved population after the 11 September 2001 attack in New York promoted the creation of a broad range of group interventions with children and their parents using inventive activities, rituals and exercises to address the reconciliation and reconstitution processes of children at different cognitive and emotional levels, especially during the first year after the death.

One New Jersey programme has developed a detailed manual that includes handouts, exercises and session guides. The objectives of the six sessions follow more traditional descriptions of the tasks of grief originally articulated by Worden (2002): (i) getting to know each other, (ii) living with feelings, (iii) patching memories together, (iv) reviewing the way we were and the way we are, (v) getting help from friends, and (vi) describing 'what we hold in our hearts'. Six group sessions were held separately for parents and for five different developmental age groups (3, 4–5, 6–10, 11–13 and 14–16 years). Following these sessions, families were offered booster sessions at times of anniversaries, Mother's Day, Father's Day and other holidays to reflect the awareness that intense feelings of grief may resurface on occasions celebrating the family.

The following questions emerging from current research on interventions with bereaved children are discussed in this chapter:

- Can ecological multisystemic approaches improve understanding of the interaction of stresses at different levels of social organization?
- Are assessments of symptoms of traumatic stress essential for bereavement interventions?
- What is the role of qualitative methods in research on childhood bereavement?
- Should intervention models change in duration, intensity and complexity?

In addition, five interventions with different populations of bereaved children have been evaluated since 1991. The findings as well as the directions these findings suggest for research practice models are reviewed later in the chapter.

Can ecological, multisystemic approaches improve understanding

Current evaluations of both practice and research in bereavement have recognized a failure to integrate social and functional aspects of the bereavement experience into practice models although the influence of external factors often is evident (Lutzke et al. 1997; Tremblay and Israel 1998; Bonanno 2001; Bonanno and Kaltman 2001). As part of the effort to broaden the understanding of grief and mourning, dual process models have been developed for both clinical practice and research in adult bereavement. These models encourage a focus that goes beyond the intrapsychic aspects of grief towards a more comprehensive view of the social and functional processes that contribute to greater variation in people's experiences of grief than is commonly understood. For example, Stroebe and Schut (1999) suggested a dual process model of bereavement consisting of (i) loss-oriented processes that include intrusion of grief, breaking of bonds with or relocation of the deceased in memory, denial or avoidance of change, and (ii) restoration-oriented processes that include attending to life changes, involvement in new things, distraction from grief, denial or avoidance, and development of new roles, identities and relationships. An 'oscillation' between these two processes is believed to reflect optimal coping.

Rubin (1999) described a two-track multidimensional model of bereavement based on his work with adults who had lost a child. The model looked separately at the child–parent relationship in the child's memory and the surviving parent's current functioning.

Christ (2000) proposed a two-dimensional model of childhood bereavement that incorporates both an ecological and a developmental dimension. Both dimensions are crucial to understanding bereaved children's behaviour and to creating relevant interventions. The two dimensions include reconciliation (referring to the internal mourning process) and reconstitution (referring to children's return to pre-death levels of functioning in multiple domains). Reconstitution also includes children's ability to create a satisfactory life experience without the lost parent's day-to-day presence.

We are proposing an ecological systems dimension to expand the perspective on bereavement beyond the exclusive focus on internal, individual psychological processes. Our project with the families of firefighters who died in the World Trade Center on 11 September 2001 provides a vivid illustration of the impact a parent's death has on family functioning while the family is being affected by other events at many different levels of social organization. As the following excerpt illustrates, these events affected the firefighters' children and wives in fundamentally important ways:

The stresses on families caused by the traumatic loss of a firefighter father were compounded by the fact that the loss was a highly public loss as well. The event itself transformed the family and each individual in it, the hook-and-ladder or engine company the father was in, the New York Fire Department (FDNY) as a paramilitary organization, and the identity of the surviving firefighters who lost 343 comrades. This event was followed by increases in marital and family stress, early retirements and health problems after working at the site to recover bodies. At the same time, firefighters became national heroes, and the dead were honoured at multiple memorials and by having streets named after them. The event transformed public perceptions of New York City into a city able to survive and live with major loss and ongoing threat, and its mayor, Rudolph Giuliani, emerged as an internationally renowned figure. The event also transformed the nation: the general public experienced collective grief and a new sense of vulnerability and the leadership developed a mission of retribution and a focus on combating terrorist threats. Finally, the event transformed the world, which had to cope with the realization that the superpower was vulnerable and thus deserved concern and support.

This highly public event further illustrates the fact that the grief experience is affected by a broad range of other changes that have occurred as a result of the loss itself as well as the profound ecological changes associated with it. Hence, the needs for support may be experienced at many different levels of social organization and may be addressed most helpfully at these different levels and at different points in time. The following excerpt is an example of the 'intertwining' of needs and responses at different levels of the system:

At the first anniversary after the World Trade Center disaster, many memorials were designed for families of firefighters who had died. That firefighters attend funerals and memorial services for fallen comrades is an important code in the Fire Department. The widows tried to fulfil their husband's obligation by attending all memorials – at least those of their husband's engine or hook-and-ladder company. However, the number became excessive and emotionally overwhelmed many families. In addition, some memorials were 'made for TV' in an effort to engage the public, but also to serve political goals rather than having a time frame and content appropriate to the needs of widows and their children. Although the families were grateful for the recognition of their loved one's heroism, many children became angry and overwhelmed by the sustained focus on intense emotions. Subsequently, widows described being 'brought down too low for too long' by sequential evocative ceremonies. Some children, especially adolescents, said, 'We don't want to be 9/11 kids any more; we just want to be kids.' As a consequence, plans for the second anniversary were scaled back markedly, with the emphasis on 'personal and private'.

Should symptoms of traumatic stress be a focus of interventions?

Although most assessments of bereaved children have not included symptoms of traumatic stress, recent reports of these symptoms as a component of some children's responses to loss have made them a necessary part of grief assessment and intervention. The study of trauma and grief emerged from different practice experiences and theoretical frameworks. Only in the past two decades have the simultaneous constellations of trauma and symptoms of grief been identified as a risk factor for longer-term adverse outcomes (Eth and Pynoos 1985; Pynoos et al. 1991; Nader 1997; Pfefferbaum et al. 1999; Cohen et al. 2002).

The proposed diagnosis of traumatic grief in children indicates that symptoms of trauma interfere with their grief. For example, remembering the lost person generates intense feelings of terror; consequently, helpful reminiscing is avoided. In this way, images of a gruesome or violent death may interfere with more positive memories. Conversely, feeling frightened and vulnerable also can elicit grief as children remember the strong caregiver who is no longer available to protect them.

'Traumatic grief' has been used to refer to conditions in children that manifest consequences of both grief and trauma (Bonanno 2001; Cohen *et al.* 2002). Investigators suggest that when symptoms of trauma and bereavement are present at the same time, it is advisable, and often essential, to address and at least partially resolve the symptoms of trauma before the bereavement issues can be processed successfully (Pynoos and Nader 1990; Figley 1996; Nader 1997; Cohen *et al.* 2001, 2002). This is now being questioned by more recent findings. The presence of symptoms of trauma may not interfere with the child's ability to grieve. In Pfeffer *et al.*'s (2002) study of children whose parent or sibling committed suicide, the children's depressive symptoms were not prolonged by the presence of symptoms of trauma. Preliminary evidence from our work with the families of New York City firefighters who died suggests that because the two constellations of symptoms are often intertwined in children, the two may need to be treated simultaneously.

Finally, current studies of traumatic grief responses in children and adolescents are exploring therapeutic approaches that will lead to the resolution of manifestations of both trauma and grief (Nader 1997; Pynoos *et al.* 1998; Cohen *et al.* 2001, 2002). An important first step in reaching this goal is to identify the presence and intensity of these responses. The Expanded Grief Inventory, developed by Layne and associates (2001) at the University of California at Los Angeles, is a measure that, in our experience, shows great promise because it categorizes the components of the traumatic grief experience as uncomplicated grief, complicated grief and traumatic responses to the death of a loved one.

What is the role of qualitative methods in bereavement research?

An important methodological development over the past decade has been the inclusion of more systematic and sophisticated qualitative strategies used in research with specific sub-populations of bereaved children to increase understanding of variations among subgroups, contextual variables and bereaved children's thought processes. To identify patterns of responses to loss and to adjust interventions accordingly, these strategies include grouping children on the basis of their developmental attributes rather than arbitrary age-related categories (Christ 2000). Other important subgroups of children include those who experienced an expected versus unexpected death; a death by suicide or homicide; the death of a parent or sibling, a public catastrophic death, such as occurred on 11 September

2001; and multiple terrorist events in affected countries. Such methods hold promise for moving the field to a new level of understanding: one that integrates population-based mediating variables with how those variables interact to affect individual outcomes differentially. Because qualitative methods can also be used to explore the total ecological context in which death occurs, they make it possible to address questions about complex situations, such as the need for intervention as stresses are occurring and at different levels of social organization: individual, family, school, community and larger governmental structures.

Should intervention models change in duration, intensity and complexity?

Increasingly, studies have concluded that recovering from grief is often a longer and more varied process for both children and adults than is commonly understood in western culture. With adequate resources and social support, the majority of bereaved children demonstrate few negative mental health outcomes in the short run – 14 months to 2 years after the death of a parent (Siegel *et al.* 1992, 1996b; Fristad *et al.* 1993; Worden 1996). However, three studies have reported an increase in children's symptoms and problem behaviours after two years, highlighting the need for longer-term research to understand more fully possible delayed reactions and the influence of loss on children's functioning over the course of development (Worden 1996; Rotheram-Borus *et al.* 2003; Sandler *et al.* 2003b). For some children, each new stress may exacerbate, in a cascading fashion, previous levels of stress and perceptions of vulnerability that overwhelms their capacity to cope. Certainly, children and adolescents living in high-crime environments are more likely to experience multiple and overwhelming traumatic stresses. For all children, new, more sophisticated developmental abilities and added developmental, cultural–ecological demands have the potential to evoke the memory and the grief of previous losses in new ways as they mature.

A 16-year-old girl whose firefighter father died during the attack on the World Trade Center when she was 14 years of age had managed the first two years of bereavement with extraordinary resilience. She received excellent grades, spoke openly about her grief, maintained her hobbies and friendships, and began planning for college. However, the second anniversary of her father's death was shortly followed by her Sweet 16 birthday. For months leading up to her birthday – in addition to participating in memorials for her father – she attended the birthdays of friends and watched them dance with their fathers.

As her birthday approached she became acutely depressed and withdrawn and found school overwhelming. She thought she must be crazy to respond that way two years after her father's death. However, her developmentally normal, gradual separation from her mother had been delayed because of the traumatic loss. A sequence of reminders, occurrences, and cognitive and psychological changes led her to experience a transient depression associated with feelings of abandonment. When she understood that her acute depressive reaction would be time limited, was perfectly normal and expected, and was her response to the multiple external stresses, she creatively decided to do something different from her peers for her birthday. She went with a small group of friends to a Broadway musical that was full of dancing, her favourite hobby.

What remains unclear is whether and how losing a parent in childhood may create a greater vulnerability to later life events and transitions. In which children does the death increase negative expectations and intense feelings of hopelessness and helplessness in the face of stressful situations or reminders of the loss? Conversely, which children are likely to develop greater confidence in their ability to cope with stress as they master successive related challenges?

The world changes dramatically for most children after a parent's death, whether the death was the result of illness or an unexpected and traumatic occurrence. Multiple other changes take place that may only become apparent to the children over time. Their surviving parent may become depressed or unable to help them learn and develop, as the parent who died was able to do. They may have to move from the family home. They are faced with constant reminders of something missing in their lives: the guidance, support, affection and strength formerly provided by the lost parent. Therefore, interventions need to focus not only on helping children with their grief over the lost relationship and the lost parent's specific functions but over the secondary changes that are a consequence of the death as well.

Ryan, aged 13 years, became acutely depressed, with suicidal thoughts, 18 months after his firefighter father died. His mother requested crisis intervention from our FDNY Family Assessment and Guidance Program. Ryan was a good student, but his grades had dipped during the year after his father's death. Thus, it was uncertain whether the high school his father and uncles had attended would accept him. Ryan tearfully said that he felt dumb because his grades were down a level from what they had been before the death. He found a tutor, and his grades began to improve, but it was taking time. He found he was unable to retain information and think clearly during tests, although he had studied. Our intervention focused on normalizing his drop in grades and his test anxiety and supported his need for more time to recover from the severe loss. It also supported his mother in her anger at the school's insensitivity. We emphasized that her son's psychological distress was likely to be transient in nature. Although we offered his mother advocacy, she wanted to try to prevail with the school on her own. When the high school notified Ryan that he had been accepted, his grades rapidly improved and his test anxiety disappeared.

Practice models may require a paradigmatic change from the more traditional focus on a specific time-limited package of interventions with specific individual, family and group therapies to a model that incorporates the total ecological context over a longer period. Researchers have suggested that this new paradigm is a way to make services more accessible and acceptable to clients (Duan and Rotheram-Borus 1999; Jordan and Neimeyer 2003; Leonard et al. 2003; Rotheram-Borus and Duan 2003; Rotheram-Borus et al. 2003). The paradigm also may include participation in multiple interventions simultaneously.

Formally evaluated child bereavement interventions

Over the past two decades, five interventions for bereaved children have used comparison groups to test the effectiveness of such interventions. These interventions are based on research that compared parentally bereaved children and non-bereaved children and found that parentally bereaved children had significantly more psychosocial problems, including anxiety and depression (Weller et al. 1991; Siegel et al. 1996a; Dowdney 2000). These findings and their implications for practice and research are reviewed briefly below.

Two of the five studies began after a parent's anticipated or sudden death; the third study began after the suicide of a sibling or parent. The other two studies began during a parent's terminal illness from cancer or from AIDS and included follow-up from one to four years. The interventions were based on cognitive behavioural, psycho-educational and supportive theories. Three used parallel parent and child group interventions, and two used individual family-focused approaches (see Table 7.1, pp. 106–7).

A home-based family intervention

Black and Urbanowicz (1985, 1987) evaluated an intervention offered to 46 families with children younger than 16 years after one parent died. The intervention consisted of six home-based family counselling sessions beginning approximately two months after the parent's death. Sessions were planned to provide emotional support, help with problem-solving, encourage communication about the dead parent, and facilitate the expression and resolution of grief. Of the 46 families offered the intervention, 33 entered the study and 22 completed four to six sessions. The control group consisted of 34 bereaved families that were contacted for the first time a year after the death. The investigators were psychiatric social workers with specialized training in bereavement counselling.

A follow-up evaluation that included a structured interview was completed a year after the death and again two years later. Relying exclusively on parents' reports, the investigators found that children whose families had participated in the treatment group had fewer behavioural and learning problems and a lower incidence of depression and sleep or health problems. They also found that children in the treatment group spent more time talking and crying about the dead parent and that crying was associated with fewer, less serious behavioural problems, especially among children older than 5 years. At the two-year follow-up, the investigators reported trends towards greater improvement in the treatment groups but no significant outcomes on mental health assessments. They reported difficulty in obtaining evaluations from the control group. Its exclusive reliance on parents' reports and the lack of details about the content of the intervention have been identified as limitations of this early study (Tremblay and Israel 1998).

A family bereavement group programme

Sandler and associates (Sandler *et al.* 2003a,b) studied a cognitive behavioural intervention at the Prevention Research Center, Arizona State University, funded by the National Institute of Mental Health. The intervention was based on their previously tested interventions with divorced families. The intervention tested the efficacy of approaches involving training in parenting skills to reduce stress and to build the coping capacities of bereaved children and parents. It was delivered in 11 group sessions with bereaved parents and 11 parallel group sessions with the children. Ninety families (135 children and adolescents and their caregivers) were randomly assigned to the intervention, and 66 families (109 children and their caregivers) were assigned to a comparison group involving self-study with printed materials.

All the families were referred to the bereavement programme by family service, health and mental health agencies that were providing mental health services to the families. Sandler and associates suggest that their method of accrual may have accounted for the greater numbers of mental health problems reported when the study began than has been found in other child bereavement studies (Sandler *et al.* 2003b). For example, 41 per cent of the children in their study had clinically significant problems

Table 7.1   Formally evaluated childhood bereavement interventions

	Black and Urbanowicz (1987)	Sandler et al. (2003a)	Pfeffer et al. (2002)	Christ et al. (forthcoming)	Rotheram-Borus et al. (2003)
Population	Bereaved families with young children beginning 2 months after parent death	Bereaved families seeking mental health intervention 10 months on average after parent death (range 3–29 months)	Bereaved families in which either parent or sibling committed suicide. Began within 1 year after the death	Began with families 3–6 months before one parent died of cancer and followed 14 months after death occurred	Began with inner-city adolescents and their parents during the parent's HIV terminal illness and followed 2 years plus
Intervention approach	Supportive intervention conducted with family to promote mourning of parent and child and improve communication about the death	Cognitive behavioural parenting skills training groups to reduce stress and build coping capacities in parents and children	Psycho-educational and supportive groups for parents and children	Psycho-educational and supportive parent/child guidance to improve parent's communication, competence and consistency with children	Cognitive behavioural parent and adolescent coping skills training to reduce emotional distress, problem behaviours and teenage parenthood
Intervention format	6 home-based family counselling sessions, 2–3 weeks apart	11 parallel group sessions with bereaved parents and their children	Ten-week 1.5 hour parallel group programme for parents and children	In pre-death 3–5 and in post-death 4–6 family sessions conducted mostly in home. Evaluations at baseline and 6–14 months post-death	24 group sessions with parents and 12 with adolescents

Sample size	21 bereaved families with 38 young children	90 families with 135 children and their carers	27 families and 39 children	104 families completed intervention; 79 completed first and second evaluations	154 inner-city parents with HIV and 207 adolescents. Only 70 parents died by fourth-year follow-up
Comparison group	Families contacted for the first time 1 year after the death were the comparison group	A randomly assigned self-study comparison group given written material	A no-treatment randomly assigned comparison group (74% dropout rate)	Two comparison groups: randomly assigned telephone intervention group and school-based non-bereaved comparison group	Equal numbers of families and adolescents randomized to standard treatment group
Results	At 1 year tx group functioned better in behaviour, mood and general health although not statistically significant. Difference were attenuated at 2 years	Greater decrease in anxiety and depression in tx group. Girls and more symptomatic children at baseline benefited most. Mediating factors were identified	Greater reduction in anxiety and depression, especially with those presenting with clinical levels at baseline	Programme goals were achieved: children's evaluation of parent's competence and ability to communicate improved and was sustained 7–14 months after death	Greater decrease in emotional distress, conduct problems, multiple problem behaviours at 2 years in tx group. Most of these benefits eroded over 4 years. Still had fewer teen pregnancies

reported on the Child Behaviour Checklist, as opposed to 19 per cent of the children in the bereavement study conducted at Harvard University (Worden 1996).

Unique to this cognitive behavioural approach was the opportunity for participants to practise skills in groups with peers before applying the skills at home. The manual-based treatment groups for parents aimed to modify identified mediators of positive mental health outcomes for children who had suffered a major loss: for example, by establishing positive parent–child relationships; stable, positive routines; and effective discipline. Another goal was to protect children from life-event stressors associated with the loss of a parent. To accomplish this goal, the investigators taught parents ways to develop positive family activities; improve their listening skills; increase the warmth of family relationships; reduce negative stressors, such as family conflict and parental depression; develop clear expectations and reasonable consequences when expectations were not met (improving discipline); and challenge negative thinking by using positive reframing. The group leaders found that in each session, bereaved parents needed to discuss their own grief process in addition to parenting skills. On the basis of reliable and valid measures of the programme's constructs as well as measures of anxiety, depression and behaviour, the investigators found that the intervention improved the parents' parenting skills and coping, reduced their stress associated with events, improved their ability to express feelings and improved their mental health.

The skills taught to children and adolescents complemented the skills taught to the surviving parents. Dividing the children into two age groups (7–11 and 12–17 years), the investigators aimed to increase the children's sense of control and self-esteem, reduce their negative self-appraisals, and improve their capacity to recognize and express their feelings. At the 11-month evaluation, children exhibited fewer symptoms of anxiety and depression and less externalizing of problems, such as acting out, than did children in the comparison group. However, the effects of the intervention were not uniform across all children in the treatment groups. Those who had more severe problems before they entered the programme – especially anxiety and depression – experienced greater improvement, and girls exhibited more beneficial effects than did boys. Differences between the treatment and comparison groups had declined by the two-year follow-up.

Mediators of the intervention process included (i) improving the parents' warmth and discipline, (ii) reducing the stress associated with events the children were exposed to, and (iii) reducing the children's need to inhibit expression of their feelings.

A family intervention after a parent's or sibling's suicide

Pfeffer and colleagues (2002) conducted a 10-week, 90-minute, parallel group programme for parents and children in families where either a parent or sibling had committed suicide. Twenty-seven families with 39 children were randomly assigned to the intervention group, and 25 families with 36 children were assigned to a no-treatment comparison group. The researchers developed a manual to implement the programme using a psycho-educational and supportive group approach.

For the children, the psycho-educational components of the programme focused on understanding death and its permanence, identifying feelings of grief, defining what suicide is, discussing why people commit suicide, and enhancing the children's problem-solving skills. The aim of the supportive components was to facilitate the children's expressions of grief and identification with the positive attributes of the dead family member while avoiding suicidal urges and hopelessness. The children were encouraged to feel more optimistic, to manage traumatic thoughts and stigmatizing concerns about the suicide, and to develop new supportive relationships.

For the parents, the goals of the intervention were to increase their understanding of childhood bereavement, foster the children's expressions of grief, discuss the suicide, identify the children's negative and symptomatic reactions, and promote the children's emotional and social functioning. Although the parents received support for expressing their grief, the primary focus was strengthening their parental role.

Reduction of anxiety and depressive symptoms was significantly greater among children who received the intervention than among those who did not. However, the greatest change occurred in children with clinically significant depression when the study began. The fact that 75 per cent of the children in the comparison group dropped out of the study, whereas only 18 per cent in the intervention group did so, led to an imbalance in retention of participants in the two groups. The authors concluded that bereavement-group interventions focused on reactions to death and suicide and on improvement of coping skills can reduce the distress of children who are bereaved after a parent or sibling's suicide. Of interest was the observation that the children's symptoms of trauma and problems in social adjustment persisted despite reduced anxiety and depression. Finally, the study confirmed a finding from a study conducted at the Memorial Sloan-Kettering Cancer Center (MSKCC) (Siegel et al. 1990; Christ et al. forthcoming). Younger school-age children and early adolescents experienced higher levels of distress than did other age groups.

Interventions spanning the parent's terminal illness and after-death follow-up

Two studies initiated an intervention before the parent's death. Both studies developed ways to help families manage a parent's terminal illness at a time when they were most accessible to preventive interventions in parallel with the dying parent's intensive medical care (Rotheram-Borus 1997; Christ *et al.* forthcoming). One study targeted children whose parent was ill with, then died of, cancer; the other targeted children whose parent was diagnosed with human immunodeficiency virus (HIV).

An intervention during a parent's terminal illness with cancer

The MSKCC Child Bereavement study consisted of a supportive and psycho-educational parent–child guidance (experimental) intervention and a telephone monitoring (comparison) intervention (Siegel *et al.* 1990; Christ *et al.* forthcoming). The unique features of the study were (i) its focus on cancer deaths rather than on sudden or traumatic deaths, (ii) its initiation before the parent's death so that children's anticipatory responses could be addressed and families could be helped during this difficult period, and (iii) its use of three groups for purposes of comparison. One group consisted of bereaved families that received the intervention, the second group consisted of non-bereaved families, and the third group received a telephone support intervention designed to ensure that families received all available services, including standard social work services, provided by the hospital and the community.

The non-bereaved group consisted of 556 children ranging in age from 7 to 17 years from 434 families in the community. This group permitted a group match with children in the intervention and comparison group with regard to age, gender, number of children in the household, and family income.

The decision to begin the interventions during the parent's terminal illness was based on clinical experience indicating that the responses of family members during the terminal illness and after the death differed substantially. This clinical experience was confirmed by the finding that children in both intervention groups were significantly more anxious and depressed during the parent's terminal illness than the non-bereaved comparison group – levels of anxiety and depression that declined in both intervention groups at the 7- and 14-month follow-ups after the death (Siegel *et al.* 1992, 1996b).

The aim of the intervention was to improve the children's adjustment to the loss by enhancing the surviving parents' ability to (i) sustain their competence in providing the children with support and care after the intervention, (ii) provide the children with an environment in which they could express painful or conflicting feelings, thoughts and fantasies about the loss, and (iii) maintain consistency and stability in the children's environment. Parents were provided with the support, knowledge and insight that would enable them to promote conditions fostering the children's necessary grief work and resolution of the loss. To enhance the parents' capacity to function effectively during the family crisis, the investigators supported them in their own necessary grief work.

The number of families that completed the experimental intervention totalled 104, and 79 families completed either the first and second psychological evaluations or all three evaluations. The experimental intervention spanned approximately 12 months and included six or more 60- to 90-minute therapeutic interviews during the terminal stage of the illness and six or more interviews after the death.

The experimental intervention was effective in achieving the programme goals: it improved the children's views of the surviving parent's competence and ability to communicate with them. The children gave their parents higher ratings on parenting competence seven months after the intervention than they did after two months.

The telephone monitoring intervention was less effective. The children gave their parents lower ratings than children in the other group did two months after the intervention ended, and their ratings were even lower at seven months.

The children in both intervention groups experienced reduced anxiety and depression and their self-esteem improved between the period before and after the death. The overall similarity in mental health outcomes of scores on depression, anxiety and self-esteem of children participating in both interventions suggests that even limited interventions, such as telephone monitoring, can be helpful to families undergoing such a crisis. On a programme satisfaction questionnaire administered after completion of the intervention study, most parents indicated that they valued the help they had received, but many recommended longer-term contact with professionals and more frequent therapeutic contact with children.

A group intervention with adolescents after a parent contracted HIV

Rotheram-Borus and colleagues (2003) evaluated an intensive manual-based training intervention involving cognitive behavioural coping skills with inner-city parents diagnosed with HIV and 412 adolescent children. The goal was to improve behavioural and mental health outcomes of adolescents and parents. At the time, all participants were receiving comprehensive services from the New York City Human Resources Department's Division of AIDS Services. The adolescents were randomly assigned to either the training intervention or to standard care provided by this agency.

The group intervention consisted of two modules: one group was composed of infected parents; the other of parents and adolescents who met both separately and together. The principles of cognitive behaviour were used in the first group to improve parents' ability to cope with their seropositive status and ongoing illness-related stressors, help them with issues regarding disclosure of their status, and facilitate their ability to maintain positive family routines.

The parents in the second group focused on developing plans for custody of their children and reducing their own risky behaviours. The goals of the adolescent groups were to reduce risk-taking behaviours, adapt to the parent's illness and improve relationships. For example, the parents and adolescents participated in activities designed to help them understand how HIV had influenced their social roles, to develop skills in conflict resolution and to establish daily routines.

Over two years, the intervention demonstrated positive results in reducing the parents' and adolescents' behaviour problems and emotional distress. Adolescents who participated in the intervention reported fewer multiple behaviour problems, including number of sexual partners, cigarette smoking, frequency of alcohol use, thefts, and aggressive and criminal behaviours. Parents showed similar rates of decline in emotional distress and behaviour problems and increased self-esteem. Both parents and adolescents exhibited a more rapid decrease in distress compared with participants in the standard care intervention. After two years of the programme, 65 per cent of the parents were alive because of the effectiveness of newly developed antiretroviral therapies.

On follow-up, 24 to 28 months after recruitment, the positive effects of the intervention on the adolescents eroded, as evidenced by multiple behaviour problems and reduced self-esteem as well as more emotional distress in both parents and adolescents, increased frequency of negative family events, and parents' decreased ability to take positive action and seek social support. Rotheram-Borus and colleagues (2003) concluded that the model of a 'package' of preventive interventions was insufficient to sustain its positive effects over several years, particularly when adolescents had to deal with the impact of a chronically ill parent over a long period. They suggested that ongoing support, or a maintenance programme, would be necessary for parents and adolescents in these circumstances.

Strengths and limitations of the interventions

The studies discussed here provide evidence that interventions with bereaved children can be effective in changing specific targeted behaviours in both children and parents. These behaviours also have been found to mediate psychological outcomes of bereavement. The improvements include development of parenting skills during bereavement, enhancement of children's personal efficacy in coping, reduction of parents' emotional symptoms, improvement of parent–child communication and children's perception of parenting competence, education about the nature and meaning of suicide, and reduction of behaviour problems of parents with HIV and their children.

Three of the five studies (Black and Urbanowicz 1987; Rotheram-Borus et al. 2003; Sandler et al. 2003a) also demonstrated positive changes in the mental health of participants, especially those who were extremely distressed and had behaviour problems at entrance into the studies and in females. However, after the interventions in these three studies ended, the improvement in mental health and some behaviours declined over time. As a consequence, Rotheram-Borus and colleagues have recommended planning for longer-term maintenance programmes to sustain early gains rather than planning only a targeted, time-limited 'package of interventions' (Duan and Rotheram-Borus 1999; Rotheram-Borus and Duan 2003; Rotheram Borus et al. 2003). Furthermore, a recent review of bereavement interventions for adults who have lost a close family member has concluded that less intensive programmes with longer-term formats may be more responsive to the trajectory of recovery from loss (Jordan and Neimeyer 2003).

Longer-term maintenance also may be more effective with children faced with the reality of continuing stresses caused by peers and developmental and societal challenges without the day-to-day presence of the lost parent. As their cognitive abilities increase, children struggle to integrate their new awareness of the changing impact of the loss on their lives over time. Secondary changes in the family and community caused by the parent's illness and death also may occur over time in ways that undermine children's previous developmental gains: for example, an unhappy relationship with a new caregiver or step-parent, conflicts with extended family members, or additional illness and loss in the family.

A keenly debated question among researchers and funding agencies is why positive research findings are infused so rarely into real-world mental health practice as interventions or as models of professional practice. In addition to a longer-term intervention format, Rotheram-Borus and Duan (2003) and Jensen (2003) suggest that aspects of how research in the social and behavioural sciences is conducted, limit its translation into the practice community. These limitations include lack of clarity about which aspects of the intervention are required for effective change, unreported aspects that may have affected the participants' change, lack of resources and training available to practice professionals with regard to the specific aspects of each intervention, and failure to involve practitioners during development of the intervention to ensure that the programme addresses 'real-world' conditions.

Research interventions may be difficult to apply in practice because they are so focused and because participants are asked to forgo other interventions. Recent experiences with families who lost a firefighter father in the attacks on the World Trade Center in 2001 suggest that families may need multiple interventions simultaneously as well as interventions that vary over time. In the aftermath of the catastrophe, a broad range of both private and publicly supported interventions were developed. Typically, these interventions included bereavement groups implemented for children of different ages within a variety of community agencies that used a variety of activities: for example, bereavement groups and individual counselling in schools to help children cope with the stress they experienced there; individual counselling for some mothers provided by community agencies; medication for some mothers prescribed by the family physician; widows' groups; camps and activity groups for children; and advocacy groups.

As Rotheram-Borus and Duan (2003) point out, many studies do not identify the full range of interventions used to attract and retain participants: for instance, provision of child care, case management or crisis intervention, or meals and transportation – services that may be integral to the effectiveness of the interventions. Such services have been referred to as 'recruitment or retention strategies' to maintain subjects when developing longitudinal research designs. Unfortunately, underreporting of such services can result in underestimation of the resources required to implement an intervention effectively.

Finally, the crucial ingredients required to effect change are generally unknown. To facilitate replication with different populations, some researchers have produced manuals that provide detailed descriptions of the methods and materials they use to achieve programme goals (Sandler *et al.* 1992; Rotheram-Borus 1997; Cohen *et al.* 2001; Pfeffer *et al.* 2002; Sandler *et al.* 2003a). A book about the study conducted at MSKCC describes qualitative analytical techniques detailing the experiences of and interventions with children who were at different levels of development (Christ 2000).

A frequent question for practitioners is how to modify interventions to make them acceptable, accessible and, at the same time, efficacious with the clients in their own practice settings. To achieve comparable improvement, what elements are required, at what level of intensity, and for how long? How can the intervention be modified to address the interests, abilities, resources and limitations of a given population and a particular clinical setting?

Conclusion

Research in child bereavement has expanded considerably over the past two decades. Interventions with specific populations have demonstrated effectiveness in changing targeted behaviours and in improving mental health in the short term. However, longer-term models are needed that incorporate maintenance strategies, integrate assessments for symptoms of both trauma and grief, provide clear descriptions of multiple services, deepen understanding of the mechanisms of change, and identify the resources and training required to implement interventions effectively in real-world settings.

References

Bifulco, A., Brown, G. and Harris, T. (1987) Childhood loss of a parent, lack of adequate parental care and adult depression: a replication, *Social Psychology*, 16: 187–97.

Bifulco, A., Harris, T. and Brown, G. (1992) Mourning or inadequate care? Reexamining the relationship of maternal loss in childhood with adult depression and anxiety, *Development and Psychopathology*, 4: 433–49.

Black, D. and Urbanowicz, M.A. (1985) Bereaved children – family intervention, in J.E. Stevenson (ed.) *Recent Research in Developmental Psychopathology*. Oxford: Pergamon Press, pp. 179–87.

Black, D. and Urbanowicz, M.A. (1987) Family intervention with bereaved children, *Journal of Psychology and Psychiatry*, 28: 467–76.

Bonanno, G. (2001) Grief and emotion: a social–functional perspective, in M. Stroebe, O. Hansson, W. Stroebe and H. Schut (eds) *Handbook of Bereavement Research*. Washington, DC: American Psychological Association, pp. 493–516.

Bonanno, G. and Kaltman, S. (2001) The varieties of grief experience, *Clinical Psychology Review*, 21: 705–34.

Breier, A., Kelsoe, J.R. Jr, Kirwin, P.D., Beller, S.A., Wolkowitz, O.M. and Pickar, D. (1988) Early parental loss and development of adult psychopathology, *Archives of General Psychiatry*, 45: 987–93.

Christ, G. (2000) *Healing Children's Grief: Surviving a Parent's Death from Cancer*. New York: Oxford University Press.

Christ, G., Siegel, K., Karus, D. and Christ, A. (forthcoming). Evaluation of a preventive intervention for bereaved children. *Journal of Social Work in End-of-Life and Palliative Care.*

Cohen, J., Greenberg, T., Padlo, S. *et al.* (2001) *Cognitive Behavioral Therapy for Traumatic Bereavement in Children: Treatment Manual*. Pittsburgh, PA: Center for Traumatic Stress in Children and Adolescents, Department of Psychiatry, Allegheny General Hospital.

Cohen, J., Mannarino, A., Greenberg, T., Padlo, S. and Shipley, C. (2002) Childhood traumatic grief: concepts and controversies, *Trauma, Violence and Abuse*, 3: 307–27.

Crook, T. and Eliot, J. (1980) Parental death during childhood and adult depression: a critical review of the literature, *Psychological Bulletin*, 87: 252–9.

Dowdney, L. (2000) Childhood bereavement following parental death, *Journal of Child Psychology and Psychiatry and Allied Disciplines*, 41: 819–30.

Duan, N. and Rotheram-Borus, M. (1999) Development and dissemination of successful behavioral prevention interventions: safety, innovation, essential ingredients, robustness, and marketability, in *Translating Prevention Research into Social Work Practice*. Seattle: Prevention Research Center, School of Social Work, University of Washington.

Eth, S. and Pynoos, R. (1985) Interaction of trauma and grief in childhood, in S. Eth and R. Pynoos (eds) *Post-traumatic Stress Disorder in Children*. Washington, DC: American Psychiatric Press, pp. 169–86.

Figley, C. (1996) Traumatic death: treatment implications, in K. Dolca (ed.) *Living with Grief and Sudden Loss*, pp. 91–102. Washington, DC: Hospice Foundation of America.

Fristad, M., Jedel, R., Weller, R.A. and Weller, E.B. (1993) Psychosocial functioning in children after the death of a parent, *American Journal of Psychiatry*, 150: 511–13.

Harris, T., Brown, G. and Bifulco, A. (1987) Loss of parent in childhood and adult psychiatric disorder: the role of social class position and premarital pregnancy, *Psychological Medicine*, 17: 163–83.

Jensen, P.S. (2003) Commentary: The next generation is overdue, *Journal of the American Academy of Child and Adolescent Psychiatry*, 42: 527–30.

Jordan, J. and Neimeyer, R. (2003) Does grief counseling work?, *Death Studies*, 27: 765–86.

Kranzler, E.M., Shaffer, D., Wasserman, G. and Davies, M. (1990) Early childhood bereavement, *Journal of the American Academy of Chiild and Adolescent Psychiatry*, 29: 513–20.

Layne, C., Pynoos, R., Saltzman, W., Arslanagie, B. and Black, M. (2001) Trauma/grief focused group psychotherapy: school based post-war intervention with traumatized Bosnian adolescents, *Group Dynamics: Theory, Research, and Practice*, 5(4): 277–90.

Leonard, N.R., Lester, P., Rotheram-Borus, M.J. *et al.* (2003) Successful recruitment and retention of participants in longitudinal behavioral research, *AIDS Education and Prevention*, 15: 269–81.

Lutzke, J., Ayers, T., Sandler, I. and Barr, A. (1997) Risks and interventions for the parentally bereaved child, in S. Wolchik and L. Sandler (eds) *Handbook of Children's Coping: Linking Theory and Intervention*, pp. 215–43. New York: Plenum Press.

Nader, K. (1997) Childhood traumatic loss: interaction of trauma and grief, in C. Figley, B. Bride and N. Mazza (eds) *Death and Trauma: The Traumatology of Grieving*, pp. 17–41. New York: Hamilton.

Pfeffer, C., Jiang, H. and Tatsuyuki, K. (2002) Group intervention for children bereaved by the suicide of a relative, *Journal of the American Academy of Child and Adolescent Psychiatry*, 41: 505–13.

Pfefferbaum, B., Nixon, S.J., Tucker, P.M. *et al.* (1999) Posttraumatic stress responses in bereaved children after the Oklahoma City bombing, *Journal of the American Academy of Child and Adolescent Psychiatry*, 38: 1372–9.

Punamaeki, R., Qouta, S. and El Sarraji, I. (1997) Models of traumatic experiences and children's psychological adjustment: the roles of perceived parenting and children's own resources and activity, *Child Development*, 68: 718–28.

Pynoos, R. (1992) Grief and trauma in children and adolescents, *Bereavement Care*, 11: 2–10.

Pynoos, R. and Nader, K. (1990) Children's exposure to violence and traumatic death, *Psychiatric Annals*, 20: 334–44.

Pynoos, R., Nader, K. and March, J. (1991) Post-traumatic stress disorder, in J. Weiner (ed.) *Textbook of Childhood and Adolescent Psychiatry*, pp. 339–48. Washington, DC: American Psychiatric Association.

Pynoos, R., Goenjian, A. and Steinberg, A. (1998) A public health approach to the post-disaster treatment of children and adolescents, *Child and Adolescent Psychiatric Clinics of North America*, 7: 195–210.

Raveis, V., Siegel, K. and Karus, D. (1999) Children's psychological distress following the death of a parent, *Journal of Youth and Adolescence*, 28: 165–80.

Rotheram-Borus, M. (1997) An intervention for adolescents whose parents are living with AIDS, *Clinical Child Psychology and Psychiatry*, 2: 201–19.

Rotheram-Borus, M. and Duan, N. (2003) Next generation of preventive interventions, *Journal of the American Academy of Child and Adolescent Psychiatry*, 42: 518–26.

Rotheram-Borus, M., Lee, M., Leonard, N. *et al.* (2003) Four-year behavioral outcomes of an intervention for parents living with HIV and their adolescent children, *AIDS*, 17: 1217–25.

Rubin, S. (1999) The two-track model of bereavement: overview, retrospect and prospect, *Death Studies*, 23: 681–714.

Saler, L. and Skolnick, N. (1992) Childhood parental death and depression in adulthood: roles of surviving parent and family environment, *American Journal of Orthopsychiatry*, 62: 504–16.

Sandler, L.N., West, S.G., Baca, L. *et al.* (1992) Linking empirically based theory and evaluation: the Family Bereavement Program, *American Journal of Community Psychology*, 20: 491–521.

Sandler, I., Ayers, T., Wolchik, S. *et al.* (2003a) The Family Bereavement Program: efficacy evaluation of a theory-based prevention program for parentally bereaved children and adolescents, *Journal of Consulting and Clinical Psychology*, 71: 587–600.

Sandler, I., Wolchik, S., Davis, C., Haine, R. and Ayers, T. (2003b) Correlational and experimental study of resilience for children of divorce and parentally bereaved children, in S. Luthar (ed.) *Resilience and Vulnerability: Adaptation in the Context of Childhood Adversities*, pp. 213–40. New York: Cambridge University Press.

Schaefer, E.S. (1965) Children's reports of parental behavior: an inventory, *Child Development*, 36: 413–24.

Siegel, K., Mesagno, R. and Christ, G. (1990) A preventive program for bereaved children, *American Journal of Orthopsychiatry*, 60: 168–75.

Siegel, K., Mesagno, F.P., Karus, D. *et al.* (1992) Psychosocial adjustment of children with a terminally ill parent, *Journal of the American Academy of Child and Adolescent Psychiatry*, 31: 327–33.

Siegel, K., Raveis, V. and Karus, D. (1996a) Patterns of communication with children when a parent has cancer, in C. Cooper, L. Baider and A. Kaplan De-Nour (eds) *Cancer and the Family*, pp. 109–28. New York: John Wiley.

Siegel, K., Karus, D. and Raveis, V. (1996b) Adjustment of children facing the death of a parent due to cancer, *Journal of the American Academy of Child and Adolescent Psychiatry*, 35: 442–50.

Stroebe, M. and Schut, H. (1999) The dual process model of coping with bereavement: rationale and description, *Death Studies*, 23: 197–224.

Tennant, C. (1988) Parental loss in childhood: its effect in adult life, *Archives of General Psychiatry*, 45: 1045–9.

Tennant, C., Bebbington, P. and Hurry, J. (1980) Parental death in childhood and risk of adult depressive disorders: a review, *Psychological Medicine*, 10: 289–99.

Tremblay, G.C. and Israel, A.C. (1998) Children's adjustment to parental death, *Clinical Psychology: Science and Practice*, 5: 424–38.

Van Eerdewegh, M.P., Clayton, P. and van Eerdewegh, P. (1985) The bereaved child: variables influencing early psychopathology, *British Journal of Psychiatry*, 147: 188–94.

Weller, R., Weller, E.B., Fristad, M.A. and Bowes, J.M. (1991) Depression in recently bereaved prepubertal children, *American Journal of Psychiatry*, 148: 1536–40.

Worden, W. (1996) *Children and Grief: When a Parent Dies*. New York: Guilford Press.

Worden, W. (2002) *Grief Counseling and Grief Therapy*. New York: Springer.

Involving service users in palliative care: from theory to practice

Peter Beresford, Suzy Croft, Lesley Adshead, Jean Walker and Karen Wilman

The pressures for participation

User, patient and public involvement have all gained high priority in UK public policy and services. The Calman Hine Report in 1995 paved the way for user involvement in palliative care by recommending that cancer services should be patient-centred (Department of Health 1995). The National Health Service Cancer Plan (Department of Health 2000) encourages user involvement in the context of recognizing the quality of cancer services as a national priority. There is a broader emphasis on patient/carer experiences and satisfaction with services. The UK government has established a Commission on Patient and Public Involvement for the NHS, headed by a 'participation czar'. In 2003, the government established a major NHS consultation – Choice, Responsiveness and Equity in the NHS and Social Care – which placed a specific emphasis on patient and user involvement and which directly involved service users in eight officially appointed task groups, including one focusing on long-term conditions, which addressed palliative care issues (Department of Health/NHS 2003).

These developments have taken place within a wider context of government emphasis on user involvement and service users being at the centre of health and social care services. This has encouraged the development of user groups and organizations across a wide range of health and social care service users, including, notably, disabled people, mental health service users/survivors, older people, people living with cancer, people with learning difficulties and people living with HIV/AIDS.

There are, however, some significant and interesting contradictions about user involvement in palliative care. Palliative care, notably as embodied in the hospice movement, has always emphasized the centrality of the patient or service user and its own 'holistic' approach to provision and practice. It has highlighted its concern with the individual's physical, social, psychological and spiritual needs. It has historically placed an emphasis on 'voice and choice', concepts which have subsequently gained a prominent place in the health and care lexicon. As one of the founding figures of the hospice movement, Dame Cicely Saunders said that one of its principal and explicit aims was to provide a 'voice for the voiceless' (Oliviere 2000).

Nevertheless, it can be argued that hospice and palliative care have been slow to address 'user involvement'. Except for the development of patient satisfaction surveys, whose helpfulness as a form of user involvement is open to question, it was not until the late 1990s that user involvement really emerged as an issue in palliative care, with the beginning of public discussion, organized events, publications and the commissioning of research (Beresford *et al.* 2001; National Hospice Council 2001; Oliviere 2001; Kraus *et al.* 2003; Monroe and Oliviere 2003). By contrast, user involvement was a legislative requirement in social care from the early 1990s and participatory developments in that field can be traced to the early 1980s. Similarly, schemes for user involvement in mental health services were under development from the mid-1980s, and in the field of disability from the 1970s (Campbell 1996; Campbell and Oliver 1996).

The pressures against participation

Because no research studies have been undertaken, it is possible only to speculate why hospice and palliative care may have come late to user involvement. One explanation might be the feeling that 'we are doing it anyway' – the sense that patients are involved routinely – following from the long-standing commitments in this field to listen to the patient/service user and to act as an advocate for them. However, offering a voice is not the same as accessing people's *own* voice. Another explanation may be that, while multidisciplinary and committed to a holistic way of working, palliative care has tended to be medically led. Health services more generally have been slower to address issues of participation than social care services. The latter are now acknowledged to have had a pioneering role in this field. But this still would not explain why palliative care came later to participation than some other areas of health specialism, for example mental health.

It is the third possible explanation that seems the most likely. Hospice and palliative care services work with two groups of people who are seen as particularly vulnerable in society. These are people with life-limiting illnesses who may be facing death and people who are either facing bereavement or have been bereaved. Thus palliative care service users are at very difficult times in their lives, having to cope with massive change, fears for the future and possibly financial uncertainty. For some it may mean having little time and feeling weak and very ill; for others, coping with loss and perhaps the prospect of loneliness and isolation.

It would not be surprising if workers and agencies were reluctant to place additional burdens on service users who can already be seen to have other difficulties and preoccupations. Furthermore, death, dying and loss are still areas of taboo in western societies. Workers and managers do express particular concerns about involving palliative care patients and service users. Issues are raised about how meaningful such involvement may be at the 'end-of-life stage' of people's illness. There has also been a significantly pessimistic strand in academic and research discussions of user involvement in palliative care. Fears have been raised about such involvement being stressful, unhelpful and coming to be seen as an obligation (Small and Rhodes 2000). These are important issues and need to be addressed. So far, however, they have not followed from research findings and there is no evidence base for them. Research work so far has also been based on very small numbers.

Initial experience

In contrast, where attempts have been made to involve service users with careful planning and preparation, there has been an enthusiastic response. This has included people with different conditions, who are very ill and with little time to live. There have been some significant recent developments. In 1999, a national seminar on improving quality and developing user involvement in palliative care was held (Beresford et al. 2000). This was jointly organized with current palliative care service users and attended by a majority of service users. User involvement was made the subject of the National Council Annual Awards scheme in 2001. This led to the establishment of a User Involvement Panel, hosted by Help the Hospices and composed of palliative care service users and others. The Panel developed and ran a series of educational regional seminars on user involvement, culminating in the first national conference on this subject held in 2003 (Beresford 2004).

Progress in developing user involvement in palliative care is undoubtedly being made. However, these events have also highlighted, through contact with a wide range of managers, practitioners and service users, that it is still at an early stage, patchy in implementation and raising a number of concerns and uncertainties from service providers. At the same time, most of the large, independent palliative care and related organizations, including Marie Curie, Macmillan Cancer Relief, Help the Hospices, the National Hospice Council and Sue Ryder Care, have variously developed their own policies and initiatives for user involvement. It is important at this stage neither to over- or understate the progress that has been made. What is likely to be most helpful is some critical consideration of major concerns being raised in relation to this issue. The aim in this chapter is to explore user involvement in palliative care in the broader context of theoretical and practical developments, drawing on a wider range of policy areas.

People's feelings about involvement need to be put into context. There is no question that participation can be a negative and unhelpful activity (Cooke and Kothari 2001). Arnstein's development of a ladder of participation has long highlighted this (Arnstein 1969). Her ladder descended from 'citizen power', through 'placation' to 'manipulation'. But such deficiencies are less to do with the inherent nature of participation itself and more to do with what participation constitutes and what purpose it serves in any given situation.

Palliative care service users who get involved generally seem to value the activity. However, only a small proportion of such service users have responded to invitations to get involved. But this is true of most groups – both of service users and of other people. We are likely to need to look to broader structural issues for an understanding of this, including the fact that we live in a representative, not participatory, democracy, where many people do not expect and are not accustomed to 'getting involved' in formal public policy or state-related activities.

Equally, reservations have traditionally been raised about the involvement of many 'vulnerable' groups. This has frequently been the case in relation to people with learning difficulties, particularly those seen as having 'profound' or 'multiple handicaps' or who did not communicate verbally. But there are few groups this has not been raised in relation to during the course of the modern development of participation policy and practice, including children and young people, mental health service users/survivors and others who have experienced long-term institutionalization (White *et al.* 1988; Dowson 1990; Thompson 1991). Concerns have been raised that such groups would not be able to contribute, would be liable to manipulation, be left exposed and would experience distress as a result. No body of evidence has developed to support these concerns, influential though they have been. It is helpful to recognize that they are not new issues, but have frequently been identified and applied to many groups and individuals.

Such concerns have often been associated with traditions of 'protecting' (vulnerable) service users, issues of 'gatekeeping' by service providers and paternalistic health and welfare cultures. This is in sharp contrast to more recent thinking that patients and service users should have the chance to be 'co-producers' of their own welfare. It is also now established that a wide range of groups which previously would not have been seen as able to 'get involved' have since demonstrated both their interest in being involved and the feasibility of their having an effective involvement in issues which concern them. This includes people with dementia (Allen 2001) and people with aphasia (Parr *et al.* 1998), as well as people with 'profound' learning difficulties and without verbal communication.

Prerequisites for participation

There is an important lesson here for those seeking to develop user involvement in palliative care. First, it is essential to develop relevant, helpful, appropriate and imaginative ways of involving people (Beresford and Croft 1993). As well as being clear about the nature and limits of participation on offer, it is also essential to understand how to support people's involvement effectively. Two components seem to be crucial here if people are to have a realistic chance of offering an input and exerting an influence and for this to be a positive and constructive experience. These essential components are *access* and *support*. Experience suggests that without *support*, only the most confident, well-resourced, determined and advantaged people and groups are likely to become involved. This explains the biased response that participatory initiatives have typically generated. Without *access*, efforts to become involved are likely to be arduous and ineffectual.

Access

Access includes ensuring equal access for service users to formal (and informal) decision-making structures, including those of service providers and commissioners and other relevant bodies. This includes addressing physical and wider access issues. It also means providing services which are appropriate for and match the needs of different groups, taking account of issues of diversity, particularly in relation to culture and race equality. People who do not use services are unlikely to get involved in them. It also means providing points of access which provide ongoing structured opportunities for getting involved in all aspects and layers of the organization/service. This needs to include opportunities for involvement in administrative and executive structures, including membership of relevant sub-committees, planning groups, working parties and so on. Enabling such 'cross-organizational' involvement which is truly accessible and inclusive, is likely to have major implications for the nature and structures of agencies and service providers.

Support

The need for support arises not because people lack the competence to participate in society and its organizations, but because people's participation is undermined by the dominance of certain cultures or traditions.

This is especially true for people and groups facing discrimination or who, for reasons of class, culture or restricted educational opportunity, have less power in society. Gaventa (1980) used Lukes' model of power to explain why poor Appalachian farmers in North America appeared to accept domination and oppression by huge corporations. The formal rights and channels which were open to them remained largely unused. Gaventa argued that focusing on people's apparent choices could result in ignoring the possible use of power to stifle and exclude conflict, leading to the 'victim' being blamed (on the basis of assumed 'apathy') for their non-involvement (Gaventa 1980). People may not know what is possible or how to get involved; may not like to ask for too much or they may be reluctant to complain. In addition, those facing particular barriers and difficulties may need support to enable them to reduce or remove the barriers (Campbell and Oliver 1996; Oliver 1996). There are at least five essential elements to support. These are:

- *Personal development* – to increase people's expectations, assertiveness, self-confidence and self-esteem.
- *Skill development* – to build the skills people need to participate on their own terms and to develop their own approaches to involvement.
- *Practical support* – to enable people to take part, including providing access to information, child care, transport, meeting places, advocacy, payment for costs and expertise.
- *Equal opportunities* – to ensure that everyone can take part on as equal terms as possible, ensuring the involvement of black and minority ethnic service users; service users who communicate differently, who require personal assistance, and so on.
- *Support for people to get together and work in groups* – including administrative and infrastructural support and funding; costs for user-controlled organizations, payment for workers, training, outreach and developmental costs.

Palliative care service users are likely to have a range of additional support needs. For example, in events bringing palliative care service users together, these particular needs will include:

- providing a quiet room for people to go to if they are tired or need a break (providing bed and rest chair);
- personal assistance;
- qualified nursing support;
- provision of reliable, comfortable, accessible, door-to-door transport;
- the opportunity (with support) to tape-record contributions (rather than present them directly);
- meeting costs, if necessary, of workers with whom service users are familiar, to come and provide support;

- accessible meeting places;
- short sessions, with adequate breaks;
- meeting costs in advance;
- meeting a wide range of dietary requirements.

The value base of participation

Participation, or user involvement, like all political and public policy concepts, is far from being a neutral concept. We have already touched on its progressive and regulatory potential; its capacity to tokenize as well as to empower. Neither its nature nor its purpose is fixed. Nor is there any consensus about its definition or meaning.

More than a generation ago, Arnstein laid down a marker for thinking about the *extent* of participation (Arnstein 1969). More recently, two distinct approaches to participation, based on competing ideological models, have emerged. While these models have not usually been made explicit, they have provided the basis for development across public policy, including palliative care. These two approaches can most accurately be characterized as 'managerialist/consumerist' and 'democratic' approaches to participation.

The managerialist/consumerist approach to user involvement came to prominence in the 1980s with the political right's questioning of state welfare and increased emphasis on the market. It has been the main approach to user involvement adopted by state and service system. Its progress has continued in the UK in the context of the New Labour government's 'third way' remix of state and market interventions and emphasis on managerialism. Similar developments took place under President Clinton in the USA and have subsequently been reflected in the politics of a number of European countries. Such a managerialist/consumerist approach to participation reflects the broader interest associated with the market in maximizing profitability and effectiveness and the tendency to equate the latter with the former. Framed mainly in market research terms of 'improving the product' through market testing and feedback, the managerialist/consumerist approach has mainly been based on consultative and data collection methods of involvement. Its role in improving provision on the basis of 'consumer' or 'customer' intelligence-gathering, can be readily understood. Initially, such a consumerist approach was mainly related to advancing the 'three Es' highlighted for public provision by Conservative administrations: efficiency, economy and effectiveness. Since then, its use has extended to providing data for quality measurement and regulation, including audit, standard-setting, review and inspection.

The second approach to participation, the democratic approach, has been particularly linked with organizations and movements of disabled people and other health and social care service users. It is primarily concerned with people having more say in agencies, organizations and institutions which have an impact on their lives and being able to exert more control over their lives. Service users' interest in participation has been part of broader political and social philosophies which prioritize people's inclusion, autonomy, independence and the achievement of their human and civil rights. Participation has been one expression of a commitment to 'self-advocacy'; of people being able to speak and act on their own behalf. It has also been framed primarily in terms of involvement through collective action in independent disabled people's and service users' groups and organisations (Campbell 1996; Campbell and Oliver 1996; Oliver 1996; Newnes *et al.* 2001). The democratic approach to involvement is explicitly political.

A number of differences can be identified between these two approaches to participation. The first approach generally starts with policy and the service system; the second is rooted in people's lives and their aspirations to improve the nature and conditions of their lives. Both approaches may be concerned with bringing about change and influencing what happens. However, in the managerialist/consumerist approach, the search is for external input which the initiating agencies (state, service providers or policy-makers) themselves decide what to do with. The democratic approach is concerned with ensuring that participants have the direct capacity and opportunity to make change. This latter approach highlights issues of power and the (re)distribution of power. These are not explicit concerns of the managerialist/consumerist model of involvement.

It is important to distinguish between these two approaches to user involvement and not to confuse them with each other (Beresford and Croft 1996; Barnes *et al.* 1999). They do not necessarily sit comfortably together. One is managerialist and instrumental in purpose, without any commitment to the redistribution of power or control; the other is liberatory, with a commitment to personal and political empowerment. The latter's concern is with bringing about direct change in people's lives, through collective as well as individual action. The disabled people's movement, for example, bases its approach to participation on the social model of disability, using both parliamentary and direct action to achieve change. It has prioritized the introduction of civil rights and freedom of information legislation and the provision of adequate support for organizations controlled by disabled people themselves, establishing the 'independent living' movement to ensure that disabled people can maintain control over their personal support through direct payments and self-run personal assistance schemes. While the logic of the democratic approach is for 'user-led' and 'user-controlled' services, a managerialist/consumerist approach is compatible with the retention of a provider-led approach to policy and services. If the democratic approach is explicitly political (and can expect to come in for criticism for this reason), the managerialist/consumerist approach tends to be abstracted and treated as if it were unrelated to any broader ideology or philosophy. It has become the dominant approach to user involvement in health and welfare and offers a technicist approach to data collection.

What is user involvement?

These competing approaches to user involvement not only highlight issues about the politics and purpose of participation but also raise the question, what is participation? This is a question that seems to apply particularly in the context of palliative care. The issue emerged with some intensity at the first national conference on user involvement in palliative care (Beresford 2004). A big concern in the discussion and feedback from this conference was whether 'user involvement' was sometimes being confused with 'support'. For example, some participants felt that examples of involvement presented at the conference were less about involvement than about support, with comments like:

I did not feel this session shared my understanding of user involvement.

There was a confusion all the way through between . . . support groups [and] user groups which liaise quality issues to feed into the service.

[There is] the question of what does 'user participation' mean? Mutual support, or reflecting on service provision?
(Beresford 2004: 17–18)

There was no consensus about this issue. However, these comments do raise two broader points. First, such an understanding of user involvement seems to follow more from a managerialist/consumerist model of participation, where the focus is on services and service users feeding into them. Secondly, this is in contrast to the general approach of service user movements in relation to participation. Service users have argued that the two – support in the form of self-help and mutual aid, and involvement for change – are inextricable (Oliver 1996). This is also embodied in the meanings they attach to the related concept of empowerment, which place an emphasis on both *personal* and *political* development and change (Jacks 1995).

Perhaps an important question that follows from this discussion is whether it is any longer helpful to try to distinguish between and separate 'support' and 'involvement'. Thus support groups and initiatives that do not address issues of involvement, and user involvement groups and initiatives that do not address issues of support, may both be problematical. The solution may be to ensure that each takes account of the other, although the emphasis may vary according to what service users (or indeed, service providers) want in any particular setting and it is important for this to be clear. Further thought needs to be given to this question in taking forward user involvement in palliative care, where issues of support are central to enabling effective and appropriate user involvement.

The centrality of involvement in occupational practice

The issues raised by palliative care highlight how understandings of participation may need to be reviewed. Initial government enthusiasm for participation in the 1990s focused on user involvement in service planning, management, and individual complaints and comment procedures. Palliative care highlights the importance of developing user involvement in *occupational practice*. There is a tendency to treat 'user involvement' as an add-on and to reify it as a separate activity of its own – in terms of people going to meetings, joining committees and filling in questionnaires.

But the key engagement that *all* service users have in palliative care is with the range of professionals and practitioners who work with them. It is here that user involvement should start and be supported. The particular value of this in palliative care is readily seen. It means that practice is seen as a joint venture into which the service user can feed, through expressing their views, ideas, preferences and wishes, to influence how practice is carried out and what happens to them. This is probably what 'good practice' has always been. Thus user involvement can be traced to what happens to any individual right from their first contact with the service, how responsive workers are to them and their individual needs, and how self-determining they are enabled or permitted to be. No less important, all the information gathered from these crucial individual relationships needs to be recognized as a prime data source and aggregated to develop and improve service quality and occupational practice.

Priority areas for involvement

There are also lessons to be learned from other fields about where user involvement can be most helpful and productive. The three priority areas are: (i) training and education; (ii) defining quality standards and measures; and (iii) evaluation and research.

Training and education

Training and education are seen by service user organizations to constitute one of the most effective ways of enabling service cultures to become more 'user-centred'. The new social work degree qualification offered in the UK requires user involvement in all aspects of such education, from recruitment to assessment, and this offers helpful learning for other fields (Levin 2004). There are many imaginative ways in which palliative care service users can contribute directly and indirectly to training.

Developing user-defined quality standards and measures

There is considerable government emphasis in the UK on measuring quality and on developing quality standards. These have largely been generated from the perspectives of managers, professionals and service providers. Yet service users may have different concerns and priorities. It is important and feasible for service users both to be involved in developing user-defined measures and to be involved centrally in the process of assessment (Shaping Our Lives and others 2003).

User involvement in evaluation and research

Government concern that policy and practice should be evidence-based has been accompanied by a concern, both from government and beyond, that service users' perspectives should be recognized as an important knowledge source and that service users should be involved in research to ensure it reflects and embodies their perspectives and concerns, alongside those of others. Service user researchers in related fields are also undertaking their own research which is finding new ways of accessing service user viewpoints as well as highlighting ways of linking with and improving policy and practice (Faulkner and Nicholls 1999).

Priority issues for user involvement

The location of user involvement which we have just discussed, that is to say, what aspects of policy and provision people can get involved in, is only one of four major issues to take account of if the goal is to develop a strategic approach to user involvement in palliative care. Such a coherent approach is likely to be based on prioritizing these four concerns for achieving effective user involvement. The four are:

- *Inclusion.* Service users, reflecting the slogan of the disabled people's movement, 'Nothing about us without us', are involved in all key decisions that agencies make that may have an impact on their lives (Charlton 2000).
- *Diversity. All* service users, whatever stage of their illness or condition, wherever they live, regardless of age, race, culture, sexuality, disability,

distress, sexuality, gender, have a real and equal chance to be involved in whatever ways are most helpful and appropriate for them.

- *Impact.* Involvement equals influence and really can lead to change along the lines sought by service users – it is not just seen as an isolated exercise whose benefits are restricted to 'taking part'. Service users, especially those facing major difficulties, get involved to make a difference. This must be recognized, respected and acted upon.
- *Location.* User involvement is offered where it is wanted and where it can be most helpful.

Conclusion

Addressing the above four issues systematically, as well as realistically, can provide the basis for an effective, productive and ethical approach to user involvement in palliative care. It offers the prospect of making it possible for service users who may be at one of the most difficult and demanding times of their lives, both to benefit and to contribute from their own experience and expertise.

References

Allen, K. (2001) *Communication and Consultation: Exploring Ways for Staff to Involve People with Dementia in Developing Services.* Bristol: Policy Press in association with the Joseph Rowntree Foundation.

Arnstein, S. (1969) A ladder of citizen participation in the USA, *Journal of the American Institute of Planners*, 35(4): 216–24.

Barnes, M., Harrison, S., Mort, M. and Shardlow, P. (1999) *Unequal Partners: User Groups and Community Care.* Bristol: Policy Press.

Beresford, P. (2004) *Listening to Us: User Involvement in Palliative Care. Report of the First National Conference on User Involvement in Palliative Care.* London, Help the Hospices.

Beresford, P. and Croft, S. (1993) *Citizen Involvement: A Practical Guide for Change.* Basingstoke: Macmillan.

Beresford, P. and Croft, S. (1996) The Politics of Participation, in D. Taylor (ed.) *Critical Social Policy: A Reader.* London, Sage.

Beresford, P., Broughton, F., Croft, S. *et al.* (2000) *Improving Quality, Developing User Involvement*: Middlesex, Centre for Citizen Participation, Brunel University.

Beresford, P., Croft, S. and Oliviere, D. (2001) *Our Lives, Not Our Illness: User Involvement in Palliative Care*, Briefing Paper 6. London: National Council for Hospice and Specialist Palliative Care Services.

Campbell, J. and Oliver, M. (1996) *Disability Politics: Understanding Our Past, Changing Our Future*. Basingstoke: Macmillan.

Campbell, P. (1996) The history of the user movement in the United Kingdom, in T. Heller, J. Reynolds, R. Gomm, R. Muston and S. Pattison (eds) *Mental Health Matters*. Basingstoke: Macmillan.

Charlton, J.I. (2000) *Nothing About Us Without Us: Disability, Oppression and Empowerment*. Berkeley, CA: University of California Press.

Cooke, B. and Kothari, U. (2001) *Participation: The New Tyranny?* London: Zed Books.

Department of Health (1995) *A Policy Framework for Commissioning Cancer Services. A Report by the Expert Advisory Group on Cancer to the Chief Medical Officers of England and Wales* (Calman Hine Report). London: Department of Health.

Department of Health (2000) *The National Cancer Plan*. London: Department of Health.

Department of Health/NHS (2003) *Building on the Best: Choice, Responsiveness and Equity in the NHS*, Strategy Paper. London: The Stationery Office.

Dowson, S. (1990) *Keeping It Safe: Self-advocacy by People with Learning Difficulties and the Professional Response*. London: Values Into Action.

Faulkner, A. and Nicholls, V. (1999) *The DIY Guide to Survivor Research*. London: Mental Health Foundation.

Gaventa, J. (1980) *Power and Powerlessness: Quiescence and Rebellion in an Appalachian Valley*. Oxford: Clarendon Press.

Jacks, R. (ed.) (1995) *Empowerment in Community Care*. London: Chapman & Hall.

Kraus, F., Levy, J. and Oliviere, D. (2003) Brief report on user involvement at St Christopher's Hospice, *Palliative Medicine*, 17: 375–7.

Levin, E. (2004) *Involving Service Users and Carers in the New Social Work Degree: A Resource Guide*. London: Social Care Institute for Excellence.

Monroe, B. and Oliviere, D. (2003) *Patient Participation in Palliative Care: A Voice for the Voiceless*. Oxford: Oxford University Press.

Newnes, C., Holmes, G. and Dunn, C. (eds) (2001) *This Is Madness Too: Critical Perspectives on Mental Health Services*. Ross-on-Wye: PCCS Books.

National Hospice Council (2001) Support and self-help for people with new diagnosis: user involvement, *Information Exchange* (National Hospice Council), September, p. 11.

Oliver, M. (1996) *Understanding Disability: From Theory to Practice*. Basingstoke: Macmillan.

Oliviere, D. (2000) A voice for the voiceless, *European Journal of Palliative Care*, 7(3): 102–5.

Oliviere, D. (2001) User involvement in palliative care services, *European Journal of Palliative Care*, 8(6): 238–41.

Parr, S., Byng, S., Gilpin, S. with Ireland, C. (1998) *Talking about Aphasia*. Buckingham: Open University Press.

Shaping Our Lives and others (2003) *Shaping Our Lives – From Outset to Outcome: What People Think of the Social Care Services They Use*. York: Joseph Rowntree Foundation.

Small, N. and Rhodes, P. (2000) *Too Ill to Talk? User Involvement and Palliative Care*. London: Routledge.

Thompson, C. (ed.) (1991) *Changing the Balance: Power and People who use Services*. Community Care Project, London: National Council for Voluntary Organisations.

White, I., Devenney, M., Bhaduri, R. *et al.* (eds) (1988) *Hearing the Voice of the Consumer*. London: Policy Studies Institute.

9 | Excluded and vulnerable groups of service users

Felicity Hearn

The way that western society is structured results in many people becoming marginalized, oppressed and devalued (Thompson 2002). Good practice in the field of loss and bereavement should be about recognizing these social processes and actively seeking to reduce discrimination, rather than inadvertently marginalizing or excluding people further. This chapter addresses *vulnerability* to the experience of loss and bereavement and, more particularly, *exclusion* from the receipt of palliative care and bereavement support services. This relates as much to the broad fields of health and social care, where the palliative approach is integral, as to more specific specialist teams and settings.

What is social exclusion?

Social exclusion is a complex, multidimensional concept, usefully explored in depth by Pierson (2002). In summary, it is a process including elements of discrimination and oppression, cutting people off from services, social networks and opportunities for development.

Tackling social exclusion and promoting its opposite, social inclusion, has wide political appeal, although this can mean different things to different people, those on the political left seeing it as a push towards equality and tackling deprivation, and those on the political right seeing it as a push towards a more cohesive unified society, a strong nation (Pierson 2002). A prevailing theme of this chapter is the need to interpret social inclusion more broadly than we have done previously in palliative care and bereavement services.

At its outset in the 1960s, the modern hospice movement was pioneering in addressing disadvantage even though the term 'social exclusion' emerged later, in French social policy during the 1970s, when 'Les exclus' came to refer to people living on the margins of society in France (Jordan 1997). St Christopher's Hospice, the first modern hospice in the UK, was founded in 1967 by Dame Cicely Saunders, espousing a holistic philosophy of hospitality to a varied community of people (Clark 1998). Over the past century, standards of living and quality of life have risen for many people, but substantial pockets of relative poverty remain, both financial and in terms of access to services.

Exclusion in relation to loss, dying and bereavement

People with life-threatening illnesses already face multiple losses, including the ultimate loss of life. They may additionally face exclusion by being outside the conventional social structures, for example school, work, social clubs, sometimes choosing to avoid others in a similar situation. According to one carer of a person with multiple sclerosis:

> When he was well he didn't like seeing people worse than him. Then, when he got worse, he got worse quickly and was not able to meet. He didn't get help really from others; he couldn't take part in anything. It was a huge effort in the end.
>
> (Joseph Rowntree Foundation 2002: 2)

Bereaved people may be similarly excluded from mainstream society, albeit for a temporary period. There are examples in both policy and practice of the exclusion of dying people being tackled. One notable example is the successful campaign led by the Association of Hospice and Specialist Palliative Care Social Workers, resulting in the introduction of the Special Rules for Attendance Allowance and Disability Living Allowance in 1990. Another is the development in many localities of more flexible home care support for terminally ill people. However, provision is patchy and funding often short term.

We need to critically evaluate whether members of vulnerable groups in society are excluded from loss and bereavement support services, and why. Palliative care services do not adequately reach disadvantaged groups in society as they focus on physical and psychological needs, deflecting attention from social needs (National Council of Hospice and Specialist Palliative Care Services, 2000b). As social care has been undervalued in the composite term 'psychosocial care', the National Council recommends substituting the two terms 'psychological care' and 'social care' in order to 're-emphasize the social'. Thompson (2002) asserts similarly that traditional approaches to loss and bereavement 'can be criticized for their psychological reductionism' (p. 5), as they omit the cultural dimension of shared meanings and the structural dimension of social relations. There is a need to move beyond a narrow individualistic focus to see the wider social context: power relations and the social divisions that underpin them, including race, disability, gender and sexuality.

Discrimination and exclusion become magnified when a dying or bereaved person is also a member of a stigmatized group. The complexity of addressing multiple layers of exclusion is challenging even to staff who are committed to anti-discriminatory practice. Where they are not, the issues are frequently ignored or the person is patronized. This overlap between the 'taboos' of dying and social exclusion more generally is identified in the concept of social death, defined by Sweeting and Gilhooly (1992: 251–2) as: 'the point at which a person "dies" in the social sense – the end of an individual's social identity'. People may be treated as dead before they actually are (Charmaz 1980), often on the basis of social characteristics such as old age, low economic status, learning disability or dementia.

The key principles of palliative care, namely to affirm life and to neither hasten nor postpone death, are useful guiding principles here against a societal pressure to relegate to the status of 'non-persons' people whose quality of life appears very poor. These principles are further underpinned by the Human Rights Act 1998.

Practice focus 1
An 80-year-old man was left severely mentally and physically disabled by a stroke, unable to move voluntarily, eat or speak, and cared for in a nursing home. His wife was highly distressed by his 'living death'. She struggled to accept the loss of his personality, yet continued to visit, relate to and care for him daily. The nursing home staff helped her by maintaining the man's dignity and showing his wife that they understood her profound loss. In turn, she helped the staff to continue seeing him as a person.

The modern health and social policy context

The setting up of the Social Exclusion Unit by the UK government in 1997 has encouraged policy responses to social exclusion at all levels. Oppenheim (1998) stresses the need to focus not just on those who are excluded (for example, the poor, the disadvantaged and vulnerable groups) but also on the *systems* they are excluded from. This includes hospice, specialist palliative care and bereavement support services. The Black Report (Department of Health and Social Security 1980) documented that substantial health inequalities between social classes were continuing 30 years after the foundation of the welfare state. By the 1990s, further reports on social inequalities in health were mounting up: the Acheson Inquiry (Acheson 1998) found that although death rates had fallen since the Black Report, the difference in rates between those at the top and those at the bottom of the social scale had widened. A series of National Service Frameworks and Health Improvement Programmes was commissioned in the late 1990s to monitor standards and tackle health inequalities (including the NHS Cancer Plan and *Valuing People* (Department of Health 2000, 2001)).

Nonetheless, political and policy rhetoric combating social exclusion in health care cannot eliminate discrimination. Changing practice involves a commitment to process as well as content: a change of philosophy from identifying weakness to promoting strengths, working to empower people rather than treating them as passive recipients of care. This philosophy is particularly important when people are facing major loss which threatens their sense of identity and their self-esteem.

Who may be excluded from palliative care, loss and bereavement support?

Social exclusion is clearly harder to measure than poverty alone as it is multifactorial, with different aspects working to reinforce each other. Rather than attempting to pinpoint who is excluded by whom and by how much, it is more helpful to identify social groups that are *at risk of exclusion* (see Table 9.1).

Practice focus 2

An older male traveller was dying in hospital and frequently had numerous visitors. The staff felt unsure whom to allow to stay while care was given, and how much to communicate about the prognosis to whom. They were also concerned that other patients would feel intruded upon. However, as they got to know their patient and his cultural background, staff began to understand that he viewed all his community as family. He was given a side room and family members maintained a 24-hour vigil for many days until his death.

Theoretical models relevant to exclusion in relation to loss and bereavement services

Practitioners are usually well aware of the need to treat each person as a unique individual and not to let models become prescriptive, but 'there is a world of difference between this "sitting lightly" and the practitioner who

Table 9.1   Social groups at risk of exclusion from support

Determinants of exclusion	Groups of people affected
Age	Older people Children Adolescents
Poverty and social class	On low wages On benefits Low literacy
Institutional setting	Prisoners Residents in nursing and residential care homes
Ethnicity	Minority culture groups Religious communities or groups Refugees and asylum seekers
History and social context	Travellers Prostitutes Homeless people Drug addicts
Disability	Learning disability Physical disability
Medical condition	Mental health conditions Life-limiting non-malignant conditions, e.g. heart, lung and liver failure, AIDS, cystic fibrosis Dementia
Geographical location	Developing countries Rural poverty Inner-city poverty Deprived estates
Gender and sexuality	Gay people Female carers Bereaved men

Note: These categories are not intended as boxes to fit people into. We need to avoid the dual traps of, on the one hand, treating unique people as if they are simply social categories and, on the other, failing to recognize that a person's uniqueness is shaped by their social context (Thompson 2001).

lacks any guidance other than their own presuppositions and assumptions' (Currer 2001: 23). We now consider some useful models for understanding the complexity of exclusion from loss and bereavement care.

Social model of disability

The traditional medical model sees the source of disability as the individual: the disabled person is not 'normal' and so becomes excluded (albeit unwittingly) from the mainstream. The social model, in contrast, sees the source of disability as society, the 'disabling environment'; the disabled person is not seen as abnormal; inclusion of all abilities is the goal (Oliver 1990). The attitudes underlying the social model are fundamental to modern empowering social and community work as well as to the disability movement.

Resilience model

The resilience model is not attributable to a single author, but is part of a paradigm shift of emphasis in social care and psychology from deficits or 'vulnerability to stress' to strengths or 'thriving in the face of adversity' (Seligman 1990; O'Leary 1998). The focus of attention is moved from risk factors to *protective* factors, that is, what enables people to be resilient in the face of huge challenges such as a major loss. For those who lack money and supportive family and friends, even coping with day-to-day life is an extraordinary achievement. If their strengths are recognized, people are seen as active agents, and are thereby empowered, rather than as passive victims, which is disempowering. This thinking could usefully be applied to risk assessment in bereavement, where there are tendencies both to underemphasize strengths and to give more weight to psychological than to social factors such as income and social networks.

Disenfranchised grief

Disenfranchised grief is the grief experienced when the effect of a death or other major loss on an individual is not recognized or socially supported (Doka 1999). This can happen when the *griever* is not recognized (for example, the very old, people with learning disabilities), the *loss* is not recognized (for example, a move of home, a trusted care staff member leaves), the *relationship* is not recognized (for example, an unacknowledged romantic attachment), or the *way* an individual grieves is not accepted (for example, acting-out behaviour; intense, prolonged or absent grief).

> **Practice focus 3**
>
> A 60-year-old woman with a learning disability experienced bereavement when her close friend and flatmate died. She displayed no outward signs of grief, but her support worker was concerned that she was having physical symptoms and referred her to a bereavement support group. The staff did not accept the referral, claiming that they were not skilled enough and that the other group participants might not cope with her, even though the support worker offered to accompany the woman.

Need, supply and demand model

The need, supply and demand model was developed by Smaje and Field (1997). *Need* is the ability to benefit from health care (related to both morbidity and the effectiveness of the care); *supply* is the health care that is provided; and *demand* is the health care that people ask for. These definitions are not narrowly biomedical but have neglected social and structural dimensions. The model is useful for understanding discrimination and exclusion as it provides a tool for looking at how these three fields can be made more congruent. For example, a group may be assumed not to *need* bereavement support as they do not *demand* it whereas the problem is actually that an appropriate service is not *supplied*, for example to prisoners.

To what extent people exclude themselves is an important question here. Moran and Simpkin (2000) ask if it is realistic to expect those who have been marginalized in their earlier lives to involve themselves in services that they see as irrelevant and out of touch with their lives. For example, if someone has been isolated from social contact all their life, they may not welcome attending a day hospice, particularly if there is a lack of sensitivity to their social background. People who have been disadvantaged may have low expectations of their need being met and have a greater sense of helplessness and hopelessness; Thompson (2002) terms this process 'internalizing oppression'. Nyatanga (2002) acknowledges that if culturally sensitive care is to improve, then minority ethnic groups have to become more proactive in seeking this care, and the same applies to other excluded groups. Where even one or two people from a minority start to take up a service, there is a huge incentive for 'supply' to grow and practice to improve.

> **Practice focus 4**
> A Muslim man with cancer attended his local day hospice for several months, one of the first of his community to do so. Staff and volunteers learned a great deal from him about providing appropriate care. After his death, his wife had good support from her family and local Asian community, but she also requested and benefited from seeing a bereavement support volunteer from the day hospice. Again this was a valuable learning experience for the service.

Dual process model

The dual process model, developed by Stroebe and Schut (1995), provides a structure for acknowledging practical concerns (restoration orientation) alongside emotional concerns (loss orientation). Social workers and other social care staff are directly engaged in working with people who have little power and few economic and social resources, where practical and emotional concerns are often inseparable.

> **Practice focus 5**
> A young, female east European asylum seeker received a serious cancer diagnosis after arriving in the UK. She already felt far from home, family and friends. Her considerable housing and financial difficulties were naturally compounded by her emotional distress. Partnership working between the palliative care team, the social services asylum seekers worker and a volunteer interpreter, who became a friend, provided the practical and emotional support she needed to begin to make decisions and take back some control over her situation.

Challenging exclusion of different groups

There is a paucity of research evidence on the needs and demands of excluded groups in relation to palliative care, loss and bereavement, and also on the supply of appropriate support, that is, on 'what works'. Issues *are* often being tackled at local levels, more of which need to be written up and shared. Examples of research and practice are summarized here.

Older people, including those living in residential and nursing home care

In England and Wales, 54 per cent of men and 71 per cent of women die aged 75 years or above (Office for National Statistics 1999). Deaths in old age frequently follow a longer period of dependency, involving multiple losses, and yet more attention has been paid to the loss experiences of relatively young, active, articulate people, reflecting the lower social value and status of older and disabled people. Ageism is a process that leads to trivializing the loss experiences of older people. The exclusion that results can be obvious, for example by having a maximum age for access to a service, but it can also be less visible. McLeod and Bywaters (2000) show that those over 85 years are less likely to be admitted to hospice care even though they are far more likely to be living alone.

It is estimated that over 20 per cent of people over 80 in the UK die in residential and nursing homes (Office for National Statistics 1999), so death and loss are clearly major issues for both residents and staff. Katz *et al.* (2000) point to the particular need for training in communication skills and bereavement care for these staff. In terms of bereavement support, Continuing Bonds and Meaning Construction approaches (Klass *et al.* 1996; Neimeyer 2001), which support the view that losses can be incorporated rather than 'got over', are particularly relevant to older people who are bereaved of very long-term relationships near the end of their own lives.

Practice focus 6
An 88-year-old woman who was terminally ill wanted to return home from hospital but she lived alone and her closest family member, her niece, was unable to provide any care, having other substantial caring commitments. The woman needed 24-hour nursing care and this was not available at home. She was referred to the local hospice that assessed her as needing longer-term nursing care and turned her down. She died in hospital a week later, while waiting for care funding to be agreed.

Poverty

Poverty is clearly linked to poor access to health care and low health care status (Department of Health 1999). This means that a person facing loss through their own illness or through bereavement may have already experienced many years of hardship through ill heath, unemployment, poor housing and low income. In a large-scale study of cancer deaths in England from 1985 to 1994, Higginson *et al.* (1999) identified that social deprivation is also slightly inversely correlated with death at home. Overall, 27 per cent of people died at home, but this decreased to 24 per cent in areas of high deprivation and rose to 30 per cent in areas of low deprivation. There is compelling evidence that most people would prefer to die at home (Clark and Seymour 1999), but being able to do so when community care is inadequate requires willing and available informal carers, particularly at night, or the money to pay for 24-hour care. The lack of these excludes people from a real choice to die at home. If palliative care services are to be equitable on the basis of need, these issues need to be addressed. In the UK, the New Opportunities Fund provides one source of funding for deprived areas, both rural and urban;[1] however, additional social services and continuing health care funding with clear referral criteria are required if people who are less well off are to be given the opportunity to live at home until they die.

Another important issue is the variable availability of compassionate leave from work, both to care for a family member who is dying and for the newly bereaved. Many people request sick notes from their general practitioner rather than face refusal of time off, or worse, dismissal. Statutory leave rights to provide terminal care are called for as, at present, carer's leave is not universally available.

Clark and Seymour (1999) also point to the inequity of fewer referrals to specialist palliative care services for poorer people. This may be due to a neglectful tendency to overlook poverty, or to view poor people as 'contributors to their own difficulties' (Bevan 2002: 99). In contrast, in the developing world, where poverty is widespread, hospices often direct their services at the poorest as the overall need is so great (Kornas 2002).

In a small but significant research study commissioned by Macmillan Cancer Relief, Quinn (2002) confirmed that people with cancer experienced many barriers to accessing benefit entitlements, and excluded groups disproportionately so. National and local responses in this complex field require skilled and sensitive partnerships between palliative care and benefits advice staff.

Ethnicity

Ethnicity is recognized as a major factor in social exclusion and is therefore given extended attention in Chapter 12 of this book. It should be remembered that members of minority ethnic groups often experience more than one level of exclusion. The many examples of good practice in this area include pioneering ethnic minority liaison worker posts (Jack et al. 2001) and the recent development of a series of Black and Ethnic Minority Toolkits (Macmillan Cancer Relief 2002).

Prisoners

Loss and bereavement issues for prisoners are beginning to gain attention in the UK. Potter (1999) explores the challenges for prisoners who are bereaved, whose loss is compounded by many others, including loss of freedom, home, family, social status and hope. She also highlights good practice in supporting and counselling prisoners. Prisoners are among the poorest members of society, which means they experience poorer health, and the number of terminally ill prisoners is set to increase due to longer sentences, higher imprisonment rates and the limited use of early release (Mahon 1999). One innovative aspect of the Grace Project, which works to improve end-of-life care of prisoners in the USA, is the use of volunteers from within the prison population as 'inmate hospice volunteers'. It is argued that 'no one understands a prisoner like another prisoner' and they can often take on the informal emotional support role that family members would perform at home (Ratcliff 2002: 1–2).

The issue of exclusion from mainstream hospice and palliative care has come to public attention through the case of a young man shackled to his bed until three hours before his death (Smith 1997). Debate followed over whether doctors should treat prisoners while shackled, or insist that they are unshackled. Good collaborative partnerships are emerging between hospices and the prison service, with effort being made to provide palliative care to dying prisoners which is on a par with that provided to other citizens (Oliver and Cook 1998). This is inclusive practice for a truly marginalized group.

Non-malignant conditions

Illness losses do not gain the same recognition as deaths, partly because they do not have the same rituals, so awareness of the person's grief is less (Thompson 2002). People with non-malignant conditions such as multiple sclerosis, heart failure, liver disease, lung disease, stroke and cystic fibrosis, often experience multiple losses over a longer period than people with cancer, and there are growing calls for specialist palliative care to extend its 'gold standard' of support beyond cancer to these and other life-threatening conditions not receiving the same resources (Connolly 2000). A study comparing the social care of patients with severe chronic obstructive pulmonary disease patients with inoperable lung cancer revealed that none of the former had access to specialist palliative care whereas 30 per cent of the latter did (Gore *et al.* 2000). It would be empire-building to suggest that specialist palliative care can or should take over the care of people with non-malignant conditions; rather it would be preferable to develop the palliative care skills and knowledge of staff in teams already working with patients, and offer additional specialist advice where problems arise (Chavannes 2001; Lowton 2002).

Mental illness and dementia

Another excluded group in loss and bereavement, as in society, is those with mental illness and dementia. The National Council for Hospice and Specialist Palliative Care Services report (2000a) is helpful, and again much learning can be gained through sharing case studies, for example that of a 45-year-old man with schizophrenia and lung cancer (Cabaret *et al.* 2002). The familiar issues highlighted are uncertainty of prognosis, need to stay in a familiar environment, care staff being akin to family, best-interest decisions and networking between specialist psychiatric and palliative care staff.

Learning disability

Significant progress has been made in recent years to address the palliative care and bereavement needs of this excluded group (Read 1996; Keenan and McIntosh 2000; Tuffrey-Wijne 2002). A person with a learning disability may experience loss through being seriously ill himself/herself or by having a family member or friend who is dying/has died. There are also many loss issues for family, fellow residents and day centre users and for care staff of a person with a learning disability who is terminally ill. Good practice starts with allowing people access to the same support as anyone else. In addition, useful interventions include:

- identifying past, present and anticipated future losses with the person and their family and care staff;
- developing a care plan for people with a learning disability who are diagnosed as terminally ill, such as that developed by the Mayfield Trust (2001).
- using active life-story work either as a life review (see Chapter 3 in this book) or in bereavement, including use of photos, personal possessions and visits to significant places;
- groupwork to prepare for loss and in bereavement (Persaud and Persaud 1997).

The National Network for the Palliative Care of People with Learning Disabilities has been effective in promoting and spreading good practices such as these since its formation in 1998 and is now affiliated to Help the Hospices. Local groups are active in many areas of the UK, meeting quarterly to improve collaborative work, share resources and plan education for palliative care and learning disability staff.

Practice focus 7

Sandra's story

Sandra was a woman in her forties who was born with a moderate learning disability. She lived in a succession of residential schools, hospitals and later residential homes, but still regarded her parents' house, where she latterly spent most weekends, as 'home'. Her mother recalled that, despite her disrupted life, Sandra had a great sense of humour and still managed to find things to laugh about when she was ill.

Sandra was diagnosed with breast cancer and had chemotherapy treatment by tablets. Later, while there was a major changeover of staff in her care home, with bank staff covering, she started walking less and became occasionally incontinent. Her mother sometimes found Sandra crawling on her hands and knees, and while she felt this must be due to pain, staff interpreted it as challenging behaviour. Shortly afterwards, Sandra broke her leg on standing up, and a pathological fracture due to bone secondaries was diagnosed.

On discharge from hospital, Sandra had to move to another care home as she could no longer manage stairs. A few days later, her father died. After a second hospital admission she was discharged to yet another home, and was becoming less well. When her pain and distress increased further, she was readmitted to hospital, unfortunately at a weekend when specialist palliative care was not available and achieving good pain control was a problem. Sandra's mother noted: 'It seems the medical staff didn't know how to treat her with her learning disabilities and the learning disability staff didn't know how to treat her with her physical illness.'

Sandra died in hospital a couple of days later, four years after her initial diagnosis.

Sandra's story in the Practice Focus raises a number of key learning points for challenging the exclusion of people with learning disabilities. They are, the need to:

- detect pain at an early stage;
- avoid mistaking or labelling pain as challenging behaviour;
- maintain consistency and as few changes as possible (for example, staff, accommodation);
- recognize and work with past and continuing loss issues for individuals, family and staff;
- listen and respond to emotional distress, and not label family as overprotective;

- hear the voices (verbal or non-verbal) of the person with a learning disability *and* family members who may express concerns about inadequate care, without feeling threatened;
- proactively plan collaborative working between community and hospital health and social care staff, to prevent people with learning disabilities who have palliative care needs from slipping through the net.

Sandra's close family had many issues of concern about her care throughout her illness. It was their passionate and clear perception of the gaps in her care that were the driving force in motivating staff to set up a county-wide shared training workshop for palliative care and learning disability staff to improve practice in all these areas (Hearn 2001). Following this workshop, a network group was set up to promote ongoing shared teaching, learning and collaborative working on these issues.

Conclusion

Death and bereavement threaten both our sense of coherence – what our lives mean to us – and our ability to exercise control. For groups of people who experience discrimination and hold little power, loss through death and bereavement can be compounded. Staff and volunteers who aim to support members of socially excluded groups need to recognize the difference in power held by themselves (by virtue of their professional status and role, access to resources and information) and by service users. This recognition is a prerequisite for empowering members of any vulnerable group, but is often neglected. Paradoxically, staff and volunteers feel personally and professionally power*less* when working with people from different backgrounds, and need sufficient support to reflect on issues of their own vulnerability if they are to engage with the powerlessness of service users (Gunaratnam *et al.* (1998)). It is important to remember that, 'at times, empowering the service user means defending their right to reject both the help offered and the models on which it is based' (Currer 2001: 41).

This chapter has identified a number of groups who are excluded from full access to high quality loss and bereavement services, and has outlined ways in which improvements in practice are being made in the UK. Developments in the field of people with learning disabilities have been highlighted.

Promoting the inclusion of disadvantaged groups in loss and bereavement support services is undoubtedly challenging, but it is inequitable to continue to work only with the comfortable situations with which we can easily identify. By helping vulnerable, socially excluded people to regain some control, however small, we can tackle exclusion in a tangible way.

Note

1. The New Opportunities Fund (NOF) is a National Lottery Distributor set up in 1998 to award grants to health, education and environment projects throughout the UK. Contact details: Head Office, 1 Plough Place, London EC4 1DE. Tel. 0207 211 1800, email general.enquiries@nof.org.uk

References

Acheson, D. (1998) *Independent Inquiry into Inequalities in Health: Report*. London: HMSO.

Bevan, D. (2002) Poverty and deprivation, in N. Thompson (ed.) *Loss and Grief*. Basingstoke: Palgrave.

Cabaret, W., Krerbi, Y. and Saravanne, D. (2002) Palliative care in institutions, *European Journal of Palliative Care*, 9(4): 150–2.

Charmaz, K. (1980) *The Social Reality of Death*. Reading, MA: Addison-Wesley.

Chavannes, N. (2001) A palliative approach for COPD and heart failure?, *European Journal of Palliative Care*, 8(6): 225–7.

Clark, D. (1998) Originating a movement: Cicely Saunders and the development of St Christopher's Hospice 1957–67, *Mortality*, 3(1): 43–63.

Clark, D. and Seymour, J. (1999) *Reflections on Palliative Care*. Buckingham: Open University Press.

Connolly, M. (2000) Patients with non-malignant disease deserve an equitable service, *International Journal of Palliative Nursing*, 6(2): 91–3.

Currer, C. (2001) *Responding to Grief: Dying, Bereavement and Social Care*. Basingstoke: Palgrave.

Department of Health (1999) *Saving Lives: Our Healthier Nation*, Cm. 4386. London: HMSO.

Department of Health (2000) *The NHS Cancer Plan: A Plan for Investment, A Plan for Reform*. Leeds: Department of Health.

Department of Health (2001) *Valuing People: A New Strategy Learning Disability for the 21st Century*. London: Department of Health.

Department of Health and School Security (1980) *Inequalities in Health: Report of a Research Working Group*. (The Black Report). London: DHSS.

Doka, K. (1999) Disenfranchised grief, *Bereavement Care*, 18(3): 37–9.

Gore, J., Brophy, C. and Greenstone, M. (2000) How well do we care for patients with end-stage chronic obstructive pulmonary disease?, *Thorax*, 55: 1000–6.

Gunaratnam, Y., Bremner, I., Pollock, L. and Weir, C. (1998) Anti-discrimination, emotions and professional practice, *European Journal of Palliative Care*, 5(4): 122–4.

Hearn, F. (2001) *Improving Palliative Care for People with Learning Disabilities: A Shared Training Initiative for Learning Disability and Palliative Care Staff in Gloucestershire*. Poster presented at European Congress of Palliative Care, Palermo, April 2001.

Higginson, I., Jarman, B., Astin, P. *et al.* (1999) Do social factors affect where patients die? An analysis of cancer deaths in England, *Journal of Public Health Medicine*, 21(1): 22–8.

Jack, C., Penny, L. and Nazar, W. (2001) Effective palliative care for minority ethnic groups: the role of a liaison worker, *International Journal of Palliative Nursing*, 7(8): 375–80.

Jordan, B. (1997) *A Theory of Poverty and Social Exclusion*. Cambridge: Polity Press.

Joseph Rowntree Foundation (2002) *User Involvement and the Seriously Ill*. York: Joseph Rowntree Foundation.

Katz, J., Sidell, M. and Komoramy, C. (2000) Death in homes: bereavement needs of residents, relatives and staff, *International Journal of Palliative Nursing*, 6(6): 274–9.

Keenan, P. and McIntosh, P. (2000) Learning disabilities and palliative care, *Palliative Care Today*, 9(1): 11–13.

Klass, D., Silverman, P. and Nickman, S. (1996) *Continuing Bonds: New Understandings of Grief*. London: Taylor & Francis.

Kornas, L. (2002) More than just a hospice – living with dying in Zambia, *Hospice Information Bulletin*, 1(3): 9.

Lowton, K. (2002) Can we provide effective palliative care for adults with cystic fibrosis?, *European Journal of Palliative Care*, 9(4): 142–4.

McLeod, E. and Bywaters, P. (2000) *Social Work, Health and Equality*. London: Routledge.

Macmillan Cancer Relief (2002) *The Black and Ethnic Minority Toolkit*. London: Macmillan Cancer Relief.

Mayfield Trust (2001) Policy document/care plan: Supporting a person with a life-threatening illness. Unpublished. Mayfield Trust, Gloucestershire.

Mahon, N. (1999) Death and dying behind bars – cross-cutting themes and policy imperatives, *Journal of Law, Medicine and Ethics*, 27: 213–15.

Moran, G. and Simpkin, M. (2000) Social exclusion and health, in J. Percy-Smith (ed.) *Policy Responses to Social Exclusion: Towards Inclusion?* Buckingham: Open University Press.

National Council for Hospice and Specialist Palliative Care Services (2000a) *Positive Partnerships for Adults with Severe Mental Health Problems*, Occasional Paper 17. London: NCHSPCS.

National Council for Hospice and Specialist Palliative Care Services (2000b) *What Do We Mean by Psychosocial?* Briefing 4. London: NCHSPCS.

Neimeyer, R. (2001) *Meaning Construction and the Experience of Loss*. Washington, DC: American Psychological Association.

Nyatanga, B. (2002) Culture, palliative care and multiculturalism, *International Journal of Palliative Nursing*, 8(5): 240–6.

O'Leary, V.E. (1998) Strength in the face of adversity: individual and social thriving, *Journal of Social Issues*, 54(2): 425–46.

Office for National Statistics (1999) *Mortality Statistics Registered in 1998, England and Wales*. London: HMSO.

Oliver, M. (1990) *The Politics of Disablement*. London: Macmillan.

Oliver, D. and Cook, L. (1998) The specialist palliative care of prisoners, *European Journal of Palliative Care*, 5(3): 79–80.

Oppenheim, C. (1998) *An Inclusive Society: Strategies for Tackling Poverty*. London: Institute for Public Policy Research.

Percy-Smith, J. (2000) *Policy Responses to Social Exclusion: Towards Inclusion?* Buckingham: Open University Press.

Persaud, S. and Persaud, M. (1997) Does it hurt to die? A description of bereavement work to help a group of people with learning disabilities who have suffered multiple, major losses, *Journal of Learning Disabilities for Nursing, Health and Social Care*, 1(4): 171–5.

Pierson, J. (2002) *Tackling Social Exclusion.* London: Routledge.

Potter, M. (1999) Bereavement in a prison environment, *Bereavement Care*, 18: 22–5.

Quinn, A. (2002) *Macmillan Cancer Relief Study into Benefits Advice for People with Cancer.* London: Macmillan.

Ratcliff, M. (2002) Hospice care for prisoners – the US experience, *Hospice Information Bulletin*, 1(3): 1–2.

Read, S. (1996) Helping people with learning disabilities to grieve, *British Journal of Nursing*, 5(2): 91–5.

Seligman, M.E.P. (1990) *Learned Optimism: How to Change your Mind and your Life.* New York: Simon & Schuster.

Smaje, C. and Field, D. (1997) Absent minorities? Ethnicity and the use of palliative care services, in D. Field, J. Hockey and N. Small (eds) *Death, Gender and Ethnicity.* London: Routledge.

Smith, R. (1997) Don't treat shackled patients, *British Medical Journal*, 314: 614.

Stroebe, M. and Schut, H. (1995) The dual process model of coping with loss. Paper presented at meeting of the International Work Group on Death, Dying and Bereavement, Oxford, 29 June.

Sweeting, H. and Gilhooly, M. (1992) Doctor, am I dead? A review of social death in modern societies, *Omega*, 24(4): 251–69.

Thompson, N. (2001) *Anti-discriminatory Practice.* Basingstoke: Palgrave.

Thompson, N. (2002) *Loss and Grief.* Basingstoke: Palgrave.

Tuffrey-Wijne, I. (2002) The palliative care needs of people with intellectual disabilities: a case study, *International Journal of Palliative Nursing*, 8(5): 222–32.

Richard Harding

In its definition of palliative care, the World Health Organization (WHO) states best quality of life for patients' families as an intended outcome:

> Palliative care is an approach that improves the quality of life of patients and their families facing the problems associated with life-threatening illness, through the prevention and relief of suffering by means of early identification and impeccable assessment and treatment of pain and other problems, physical, psychosocial and spiritual.
>
> (World Health Organization 2002)

In the UK, approximately 26 per cent of deaths occur at home, and over 90 per cent of patients spend the majority of their final year at home (Seale and Cartwright 1994). From 1995 to 1999, between 23.9% and 25.9% of cancer patients died at home (Office for National Statistics 2002). A UK prospective study of terminal cancer patients found that 58 per cent wished to die at home, given current circumstances, and 67 per cent would have chosen to do so if circumstances had been more favourable (Townsend *et al.* 1990). Home is clearly the preferred place of death, and changes in specialist palliative care have led to an emphasis on short-term admissions for symptom management and respite rather than long-term terminal care (Higginson 1999).

Since the inception of the modern hospice movement there has always been a strong emphasis on support for the family (Seale 1989), which would appear to be appropriate and necessary in light of the number of patients who would choose home deaths. Another UK study (Thorpe 1993) found that 23 per cent of people die at home, presenting two paradoxes: most dying people would prefer to remain at home, but most of them die in institutions, and the majority of the final year is spent at home but most people are admitted to hospital to die. The same study reviewed reasons for patient admissions, and identified strain, crisis and illness of the carer as principal reasons. Difficulties among relatives were more often cited as reasons than the difficulties of patients. Therefore, the reasons for lack of home deaths can often be seen as social and rooted in the carers (that is, informal unpaid providers of care which may be physical, psychological, emotional or practical), rather than as medical and related to the patient. Carers are faced with considerable uncertainty over the length of time they are committing themselves to care, and what may be involved in delivering that care (Payne and Ellis-Hill 2001).

This chapter starts by addressing carers in the context of UK, government health policy. It goes on to consider the challenges to professionals attempting to identify informal carers, the levels of unmet need among carers, the evidence for their effective coping strategies and resources. The current status of application of the evidence to interventions and proposed models of intervention, and the evidence for the effectiveness of such targeted services are then discussed.

Palliative care and government policy

As carers are heterogeneous, the information and support provided to them needs to be specific. The UK government recommends that people in every community need a range of support services and networks, stating that the research evidence strongly suggests that carers benefit from contact with other carers in similar situations (www.carers.gov.uk; Informal Carers, www.nationalstatistics.gov.uk). Helping carers is seen to be the best way to help the people they are caring for, and the Department of Health calls for good quality information for carers on the health needs and treatment of the patient, how to deal with the illness, and how to care.

In the past decade UK government policy has recognized the capacities of carers, and has attempted to meet their needs through the Carers (Recognition and Services) Act 1995. Department of Health guidance has set standards for quality assurance in services for carers, including the formulation of clearly defined aims and objectives, evaluation and details of how aims will be met. This Act aims to enhance existing informal support networks, and to integrate family members into service-based support. However, we lack the research evidence to tell us what the services for carers in palliative care should be, or how effective they are. Although there is frequent mention of assessment in Department of Health guidelines, interventions are rarely mentioned.

The identity of the carer in palliative care has been confused and ambiguous, but how we perceive carers is fundamental to their well-being and support (Lobchuck and Kristjanson 1997). Although hospice and palliative care services advocate a family-centred care approach, research and care services have often cast the carer in the proxy role, as a provider of information, and therefore as an extension of the patient (Neale and Clark 1992). However, the carer can be seen as holding a unique position of both providing *and* needing support, and indeed it has been suggested that it is sometimes unclear who is 'the patient' (Northouse and Peters-Golden 1993). The service conceptualization of the carer as co-worker rather than client is problematical and leaves unmet support needs (Payne *et al.* 1999). Models of supportive intervention need to carefully consider how they provide for carers, as it may not be appropriate simply to incorporate carers into existing nursing provision (Ferrell *et al.* 1995).

Formal identification of informal carers

Although the palliative care model has focused on the family, the identification of carers on behalf of services is more problematical than it may appear (Higginson 1998). A caregiver may not be actively giving care; the carer themselves may be receiving nursing care; care may be provided by more than one person; or the carer may not be a family member. Although the policy of community care underpins home palliative care, friends may be disenfranchised or excluded by professionals (Young *et al.* 1998). The difficulties faced by professionals in identifying carers are compounded by the lack of identification with the label of carer by those providing informal care (Hunt 1991). Carers are often unaware that they fit the definition of informal carer, and are unaware of their rights to assessment under the NHS and Community Care Act 1990 and of the availability of services (Henwood 1998).

A strong alliance between the family/carers and professionals has been advocated (Cull 1991). This alliance may ensure good quality care for the patient, enable the carer to take a useful role in the care of the patient (Longman *et al.* 1992), and provide the necessary support for the carer. However, these goals may be incompatible, in that carers must sometimes make decisions on behalf of patients that are detrimental to the carers themselves (Grande *et al.* 1997).

The crisis of unmet need

Carers in palliative care are seen as facing a particular set of issues, including a time-limited illness, progressive loss, the management of disclosure and awareness of disease progression, the medicalization of the home, patchy specialist services, and bereavement (Rhodes and Shaw 1999). The primary objective for many carers is to take a useful and effective role in the patient's health care, and for the patient to be comfortable (Longman *et al.* 1992). As a result of attempting to provide this care, the range of carers' consequential needs is vast, incorporating domestic help, informal support, information, and relief from fatigue, financial difficulties, anxiety and isolation (Neale 1991).

The prevalence of psychological distress and anxiety among carers of patients using home palliative care services has been demonstrated in several studies. Predictors of family anxiety in the weeks before bereavement are: being a spouse of the patient; being a patient diagnosed with breast cancer; young patient age; short time from diagnosis to death; and low patient mobility (Higginson and Priest 1996). The most severe problem identified by patients and their carers was the effect of anxiety on the family (Higginson *et al.* 1990), the authors concluding that the needs of the family may exceed those of the patient. In a study using the General Health Questionnaire (GHQ), a measure of psychological morbidity, Payne *et al.* (1999) found that 84 per cent of carers exceeded the threshold for psychological distress; younger carers had higher GHQ scores; and female carers reported higher levels of psychological distress. Increasing carer strain has been found to contribute to patient admissions (Hinton 1994).

After psychological support, information needs are second most often cited. As care and systems of delivery become increasingly complex, this need for information is unsurprising when patient management becomes palliative (Houts *et al.* 1991). A national survey of UK-based palliative care units found that only 1.5 per cent of leaflets provided for patients and families were written at the recommended level for comprehension (Payne *et al.* 2000).

Caregivers as providers of nursing care

The provision of complex nursing care, and the assessment of decisions regarding care and pain control, are important tasks in informal care. The broad range of caring tasks provided (including the administering of drugs, night care, record-keeping and fear of drug addiction), results in carers having their own specific needs. Staff must listen to carers' questions and experiences, and explain how to care (Ferell *et al.* 1991). Differences in patients' and family carers' perceptions of the experience of pain has been associated with poorer outcomes in terms of strain for both patients and carers, and the importance of effective communication and evaluation of pain by carers has been stressed (Miaskowski *et al.* 1997). Difficulties in dealing with pain for carers include fear of patients overusing drugs, drug addiction, carers having their own unmet education needs, and carers' fear of asking clinicians for pain control (Berry and Ward 1995). Studies investigating congruence of pain assessment in patient–carer dyads have found that carers rate pain more highly, and experience higher stress due to the perceived level of pain (Yeager *et al.* 1995; Kristjanson *et al.* 1998). Therefore, the provision of information and support regarding pain control may improve psychological outcomes for carers.

Effective coping resources

Coping strategies are an important area of investigation, in order both to understand who may have greatest need and to learn how to enhance existing coping through the development of interventions. For caregivers in palliative care, the period between diagnosis and death may be short, thus not allowing lengthy adjustment periods and the development of skills and coping mechanisms. In the palliative care context, although a stress response may be good if it allows the carer to cope with the situation, excessive stress negatively impacts on physical and mental health (Cull 1991). A preferred coping resource is the use of support networks (although societal changes mean that future carers may have less access to networks of support (Rhodes and Shaw 1999). A descriptive study of needs among 20 family caregivers of home hospice patients found that caregivers needed time away for themselves and for their own personal needs to be met, and that they needed adequate rest time (Steele and Fitch 1996). The use of such means of coping will often rely on there being alternative informal carers who can be called upon to provide opportunities for the carer to take a break.

The identification of effective strategies will inform the development of appropriate supportive interventions, and also enable professionals to ensure that the support offered enhances, rather than conflicts with, existing coping strategies. Finding 'windows of time', taking one day at a time, and cognitive reformulation/avoidance are noted in a qualitative study of coping strategies of informal caregivers of home hospice patients (Hull 1992). Social comparison has been reported as a useful coping strategy among cancer patients (Molleman *et al.* 1986), and this strategy has also been identified among carers of patients using palliative home care services (Hull 1992; Grande *et al.* 1997). Carers were able to benefit from the comparison of their personal caring circumstances with those of carers whom they felt were worse off in their caring situation.

Formal service support

Although various coping strategies and support networks are acknowledged, they are rarely achieved, as demonstrated in the data on unmet need. In reviewing studies of effective coping and support strategies for carers, the uptake of carer-specific services has been found to be low. In order to maximize uptake and to meet carers' needs, this reluctance to use services needs to be investigated (Hull 1992). Ensuring that there is availability is only the first step to supporting carers; we must also offer appropriate services at a pace and time that is acceptable and comfortable. It may be difficult to know when to introduce supportive services, as predicting the speed of disease progression and patients' deterioration is difficult, and there needs to be greater understanding of how patients and carers experience dilemmas in seeking or accepting help (Payne and Ellis-Hill 2001).

Outcomes that may be affected by interventions

Interventions may aim to meet the information and psychological needs described, as well as additional needs, including domestic support, respite and financial advice. Although no single intervention could meet such a broad range of needs, secondary outcomes may also be included in addition to primary intended aims. These include psychological morbidity in bereavement and grief, carers' physical health, and patient outcomes. The outcomes that may be considered by carers' interventions are both practical (for example, nursing input, information, occupational therapy aids to patient care, finance) and psycho-social (for example, support network enhancement, individual psychological support). While the amelioration in some domains may correlate with improvement in others, the intervention studies needed must articulate specific aims rather than take a 'scatter-gun' approach. Intervention studies that successfully respond to need must formulate research-based responses with specific aims if they are to be shown to be effective, and must specify the stage of caring that they aim to affect, that is, during active caring or in bereavement.

Application of evidence

There has been a considerable growth of evidence of the needs of carers in palliative care settings, demonstrating that these needs are wide-ranging and sometimes acute. These needs remain largely unmet. The research literature consistently calls for the generated evidence to be used to develop tailored interventions in order to support carers and improve their situation, and these requests for service development generally form the concluding remarks of research and review papers.

The systematic psycho-social assessment of carers in palliative care has been proposed, and comprehensive assessment schedules have been developed (Powazki and Walsh 2001). However, it is not yet clear how to meet assessed need. It appears that the development of interventions for informal caregivers in palliative care is overdue, and we need services and evaluation studies that will provide evidence of the most useful interventions (Rabins *et al.* 1990). The literature has begun to tell us who is likely to experience negative outcomes, but findings have not been systematically applied in intervention studies, and existing studies rarely pay attention to mechanisms through which interventions attain desired effects (Schulz and Quittner 1998). Important steps have been taken to apply comprehensive multidomain assessment (Etten and Kosberg 1989), but beyond the identification of specific need, we are as yet unsure as to the format and content of acceptable and effective interventions.

It has been suggested that the current lack of provision of interventions for carers amounts to a crisis approach, in that services ignore successes and reward failure (Clark 1993). Those carers who appear to be coping in their role and do not request services are assumed to have no unmet needs, and it is only in the crisis situations of imminent or apparent breakdown of the informal care situation that services respond.

Proposed models of intervention

A range of models has been proposed to meet the needs of carers in palliative care. A broad range of needs must be met, the greatest being psychological, informational and domestic; therefore a single approach will not be adequate (Hileman and Lackey 1990). The need for provision of both information and psychological support has been described. However, a study of the impact of terminal illness on spouses found that a delicate balance needs to be struck when providing new information, as this may in fact increase spouse anxiety (Willert *et al.* 1995). Information provision must distinguish between generic information and that which can only be provided by a patient's health care team (Houts *et al.* 1991). The provision of supportive interventions may be detrimental to caregivers (Siegel 1990), and this proposition has not yet been refuted due to the lack of evaluation data in services for palliative carers.

Proposed models of support need to consider acceptability in the early design stages. Studies with carers have found that self-reliance and independence are important values, despite their recognition of unmet need (Grande *et al.* 1997), and the barriers to accepting or making extensive use of services need to be more fully understood (Siegel 1990). The conflict between the need for outside help and the desire to preserve familiarity in domestic life may mean that supportive (rather than practical) services provided outside the home may be appropriate.

Home care

Home-based palliative care services usually include carer support in their aims, and generally involve home specialist nursing care that provides support for both patients and their families and carers. Carers report high satisfaction with such services (Fakhoury *et al.* 1997; Grande *et al.* 2000), describing it as useful (McMillan 1996). However, it appears that this model of intervention alone is not enough to meet the specific needs of carers. The strong evidence for high levels of unmet need reported in studies of psychological distress and unmet need in samples of home hospice informal carers demonstrates that while these services are highly valued they are not adequately meeting carers' needs.

Respite

The importance of respite services lies in providing time away from the caring role (Northouse and Peters-Golden 1993). Respite can take many forms, and may prove unacceptable to carers who are unwilling to leave the patient.

Several models have been provided. A 'sitting service' was designed to provide practical and emotional help to both cancer patients and their families, with 86 per cent of carers feeling able to leave the house when the sitter was with the patient and also valuing the opportunity to talk with the sitter (Clark *et al.* 2000). However, high costs and lack of funding opportunities for mixed health and social care interventions made the service unfeasible. A further sitting service reduced costs by the use of volunteer sitters, although issues of boundary maintenance and sitter burnout were experienced (Johnson *et al.* 1988).

Social networks and activities

An 'activation programme' for relatives of cancer patients aimed to promote an increase in active caring on behalf of carers, with the intention also of increasing social activity patterns, that is, engaging with and utilizing carers' social support and activity networks. Professional support was matched to skill increases in the carers (Haggmark *et al.* 1987). Conversely, the Well Spouse Foundation in the USA promotes the well-being of carers of the chronically ill through peer rather than professional support (Randall 1993). This national network provides telephone, postal and group support, providing information and practical sharing of ideas. The advantage of this organization is that the 'round robin' letters ensure that those who are unable to physically access services due to geographical distance are still able to access support.

One-to-one interventions

One-to-one interventions, where possible, are proposed as a means to provide carers with support and develop problem-solving and coping skills (Toseland *et al.* 1995). A cancer pain education programme has also been developed and delivered in the home for patients and carers, focusing on the management of cancer-related pain for three one-hour sessions (Ferrell *et al.* 1995). However, these interventions are time-consuming and costly, and such psychologically or individually based services may not prove to be acceptable to many carers.

Group work

Groupwork interventions in cancer and palliative care are widely suggested as an appropriate format to deliver the necessary support and information to caregivers, and similar aims have been successfully met using this format among cancer patients (Cella *et al.* 1993). Groups may be facilitated by peers or professionals, and a comparison study in gerontology between these two types of facilitation found specific benefits for each (Toseland *et al.* 1989). The peer-led group demonstrated a greater increase in use of social networks, and the professionally led group showed a greater improvement in psychological functioning.

Carers' groups may not be appropriate for all caregivers, particularly those carers who may be especially psychologically vulnerable, perhaps unable to discuss their patient or their situation without experiencing extreme distress (Ell *et al.* 1988). However, it is postulated that the benefits of requesting and giving information, sharing practical and coping skills, and social comparison processes (the comparison of one's situation with a peer group who are experiencing a similar set of circumstances) may be great (Molleman *et al.* 1986). The sharing of common experiences underpins most interventions, and other carers are seen as the most natural form of support (Slaby 1988). However, research into the effectiveness of these interventions is needed, including the format and optimum length of interventions (Holicky 1996).

Evidence of effectiveness

A systematic review reported intervention evidence for adults actively providing informal care for non-institutionalized cancer and palliative care patients (Harding and Higginson 2002). Evidence was graded according to NHS review guidelines (Cancer Guidance Sub-group of the Clinical Guidance Outcomes Group 1996), whereby strong evidence (for example from randomized controlled trials, RCTs) is graded as 1, and weak evidence (for example from cross-sectional studies) is graded as 4. Twenty-two interventions were identified, comprising home nursing care (4), respite services (3), social networks and activity enhancement (2), problem-solving and education (3), and groupwork (10). Of these, nine were delivered solely to carers (i.e. were targeted services). Only six of the carers' interventions had been evaluated, two of these had used an RCT (grades IB, i.e. strong evidence), three employed a single group methodology (two prospective grades IIIC and one retrospective grade IIIC, i.e. fairly weak evidence), and one was evaluated using facilitator feedback.

The review found a lack of outcome evaluation designs, small sample sizes and a reliance on intervention descriptions and formative evaluations. The evidence contributed more to understanding feasibility and acceptability of the various models and services (which nonetheless is very useful) than to understanding their effectiveness.

Dearth of current evidence

There is a small body of evidence on the effectiveness of interventions for carers in palliative care. There are a handful of unevaluated descriptions of interventions, which are valuable in terms of providing information about the design and format of interventions and in their description of the format and process of the intervention. They also go some way towards addressing the lack of intervention description in evaluation papers. However, evaluations, especially rigorous ones, are rare. The systematic review identified only two carer-specific (quasi-)experimental evaluations, and the feasibility of evaluation methods and the reasons for the methods chosen need to be described (Harding and Higginson 2002).

Developing interventions: steps to feasibility and effectiveness

In the light of the carers' reluctance to access services, and the dearth of effective models, the development of interventions must pay attention to key issues of feasibility (can the service be delivered?), acceptability (is the service one which carers would wish to access?), accessibility (can carers access the service should they wish to do so?) and effectiveness (are intended aims achieved?) by taking a research-based approach to design and evaluation.

An example of this approach is the 90 Minute Group, a research study that aimed to develop a research-based, short-term group intervention for informal carers of patients attending a home palliative service that is acceptable and accessible, and to evaluate it in terms of processes and outcomes for carers (Harding *et al.* 2002). The steps to achieving this were: (i) identify and review the existing evidence with regard to needs and interventions; (ii) determine carers' views on meeting their needs and accessing appropriate professional intervention; (iii) integrate findings to develop, in conjunction with clinical staff, an acceptable and accessible model of short-term group intervention; and (iv) evaluate the group in terms of uptake, processes and carer outcomes, using feasible and rigorous evaluation methods. This includes psychological measures and qualitative data collection of carers' views of benefits from attending the intervention.

The original qualitative study which informed the 90 Minute Group study aimed to investigate how carers perceived their role in relation to service access uptake and acceptability (Harding and Higginson 2001). A purposive sample of 18 carers responded to a semi-structured interview schedule. Using grounded theory, transcripts were subjected to systematic line-by-line open and axial coding. This process moved the data from categorization to conceptualization, to construct a theoretical under-standing of caregiving and appropriate professional intervention.

The central concept mediating caregivers' feelings and actions towards accessing appropriate support was found to be ambivalence. Carers rarely self-identified, and this lack of identification and recognition inhibited access to the services which they recognized as crucial sources of support. They also chose not to engage with their needs and anxieties, with a strong awareness that their choices result in the loss of life opportunities. Younger carers, in particular, reported great ambivalence about the choice between caring and other social and professional pursuits. A frequently cited barrier to professional intervention was lack of a sense of identification as credible service recipients, and caregivers were far more comfortable contacting nursing staff on behalf of the patient than for themselves. Time away from caring was the most commonly reported need, but the most difficult to meet owing to their ambivalence towards making the time. Despite strong wishes for short periods of time away from caring, they expressed unwillingness to leave the patient. Coping was primarily through distractions and activities, but these were, paradoxically, sources of distress. The need to 'escape' was complicated by the desire to remain constantly caring. A commonly reported solution was the use of 'safe' time (when a nurse or doctor was in attendance with the patient) or 'legitimate' time (for example, exercising to build up physical strength to care, going to collect a prescription). The expressed need for emotional support, particularly through talking with another, was contradicted by the use of cognitive avoidance as a means of short-term coping (by actively not thinking about the stressful situation or trigger).

Interventions for carers must consider these individuals' ambivalence. Recommendations are that the service must work with carers' lack of identification, provide safe and legitimate time and space, be time limited (that is, not add to the anxiety of being away from the patient) and be respectful of their existing coping strategies.

These key findings were combined with the findings from the systematic review (Harding and Higginson 2002) to design an intervention, providing the research basis for the development of a short-term group intervention, the 90 Minute Group (Harding *et al.* 2002). In order to ensure best care for the patient, and to reduce carers' anxiety associated with lack of information, the intervention aimed primarily to provide information. Secondly, the group aimed to provide a setting for peer exchange of information, support and coping strategies. Objectives were identified for every session, each of which contributed to the overall primary aims of the group.

The overall theme of the 90 Minute Group was *Caring for Ourselves*. This was to be achieved by combining informal teaching with group support, enabling carers to identify and strengthen their coping strategies. Multiprofessional input aimed to meet a range of needs using expert advice. Following professional input, the group processed the information in a peer setting. The group consisted of six weekly closed sessions of 90 minutes, for a maximum of 12 carers, and transport and a sitting service were provided. Each session opened with only the members and the facilitator present. Issues concerning the patient were addressed in the initial meeting before carers were asked to focus on their own needs, as patient experience of pain and symptoms have been found to be associated with carers' psychological distress (Harding *et al.* 2003). Following each invited speaker, the facilitator developed the week's topic. Directly after the close of the final session, a small party was held to mark the ending. The focus on socializing provided a positive model of ending to some difficult, and at times painful, work.

While the group was designed for carers currently caring for the patient, such work in palliative care necessarily addresses loss, change and grief. The facilitation during sessions addressed current losses for carers (and was evidenced in the ambivalence study highlighting the loss of social and career time for young carers and of a planned retirement for older carers); of change, which was addressed by carers mapping out their life balance, identifying losses and opportunities to create and guard time for themselves; and of bereavement and grief, which was noted throughout all sessions, by informational tasks such as discussing how to deal practically with death and funerals, and marking and celebrating endings through the dissolution of the group.

Uptake and process data proved the intervention to be acceptable in format and content, and outcome data demonstrate benefits gained in information, support and coping (Harding *et al.* 2004).

Conclusion

The evidence is unequivocal. Although informal carers are recognized as valid service recipients in standard definitions of palliative care, they continue to have largely unmet needs while enabling the 'good home death'. Services must ensure that good practice guidelines are clear and specific in how they conceptualize carers in relation to provision, and must make the carers' role as clients clear. Assessment must be of the carers as a distinct client from the patient, and services must provide or outsource the resources necessary to meet assessed need. This last task is complex as the evidence shows interventions for carers to be underdeveloped and largely unevaluated, and evidence has not yet been established to guide appropriate interventions for the particular needs and experiences of carers from ethnic minorities (Koffman and Higginson 2001, 2002). However, steps to feasible and acceptable intervention have been outlined, and particular attention should be paid to carers' ambivalence in order to maximize potential uptake. A further approach would be the development of meaningful user involvement to ensure that the design and delivery of interventions are in line with carers' preferences and priorities (Payne and Ellis-Hill 2001).

Any attempts to design targeted interventions for informal carers should be clear in intended objectives, and must design outcome evaluation protocols appropriate to meet stated aims. Those that aim to improve psychological morbidity should be aware that global measures of depression and burden are unlikely to show significant change. Many potential areas of need have been evidenced during the caring phases, and it is not yet known how interventions for carers currently assisting patients may affect their bereavement outcomes. However, it does appear to be appropriate and even unavoidable that interventions for carers, who actively provide informal care, address current issues of loss, bereavement and change in the palliative stages of patient management. At present, the evidence barely supports the claim that palliative care services provide effective support for informal carers.

References

Berry, P.E. and Ward, S.E. (1995) Barriers to pain management in hospice: a study of family caregivers, *Hospice Journal*, 10(4): 19–33.

Cancer Guidance Sub-group of the Clinical Guidance Outcomes Group (1996) *Improving Outcomes in Breast Cancer – The Research Evidence*. Leeds: NHS Executive.

Cella, D.F., Sarafian, B., Snider, P.A., Yellen, S.B. and Winicour, P. (1993) Evaluation of a community-based cancer support group, *Psycho-oncology*, 2: 123–32.

Clark, D. (1993) Evaluating the needs of informal carers, *Progress in Palliative Care*, 1(1): 3–5.

Clark, D., Ferguson, C. and Nelson, C. (2000) Macmillan carers schemes in England: results of a multicentre evaluation, *Palliative Medicine*, 14: 129–39.

Cull, A.M. (1991) Studying stress in care givers: art or science?, *British Journal of Cancer*, 64: 981–4.

Ell, K., Nishitimo, R., Mantell, J. and Hamovitch, M. (1988) Longitudinal analysis of psychological adaption among family members of patients with cancer, *Journal of Psychosomatic Research*, 32(4/5): 429–38.

Etten, M.J. and Kosberg, J.I. (1989) The Hospice Caregiver Assessment: a study of a case management tool for professional assistance, *Gerontologist*, 29(1): 128–31.

Fakhoury, W.K.H., McCarthy, M. and Addington-Hall, J. (1997) Carers' health status: is it associated with their evaluation of the quality of palliative care? *Scandinavian Journal of Social Medicine*, 25(4): 296–301.

Ferell, B.A., Cohen, M.Z., Rhiner, M. and Rozek, A. (1991) Pain as a metaphor for illness. Part 2: Family caregivers' management of pain, *Oncology Nursing Forum*, 18(8): 1315–21.

Ferrell, B.R., Grant, M., Chan, J., Ahn, C. and Ferell, B.A. (1995) The impact of cancer pain education on family caregivers of elderly patients, *Oncology Nursing Forum*, 22(8): 1211–18.

Grande, G.E., Todd, C.J. and Barclay, S.I.G. (1997) Support needs in the last year of life: patient and carer dilemmas, *Palliative Medicine*, 11: 202–8.

Grande, G.E., Todd, C.J., Barclay, S.I.G. and Farquhar, M.C. (2000) A randomised controlled trial of a hospital at home service for the terminally ill, *Palliative Medicine*, 14: 375–85.

Haggmark, C., Theorell, T. and Ek, B. (1987) Coping and social activity patterns among relatives of cancer patients, *Social Science and Medicine*, 25: 1021–5.

Harding, R. and Higginson, I.J. (2001) Working with ambivalence: informal carers of patients at the end of life, *Supportive Cancer Care*, 9: 642–5.

Harding, R. and Higginson, I.J. (2002) What is the best way to help caregivers in cancer and palliative care? A systematic literature review of interventions and their effectiveness, *Palliative Medicine*, 17(1): 63–71.

Harding, R., Leam, C., Pearce, A., Taylor, L. and Higginson, I.J. (2002) A multiprofessional short term group intervention for informal caregivers of patients using a home palliative care service, *Journal of Palliative Care*, 18(4): 275–81.

Harding, R., Higginson, I.J. and Donaldson, N. (2003) The relationship between patient characteristics and carer psychological status in home palliative cancer care. *Supportive Care in Cancer*, 11(10): 638–43.

Harding, R., Leam, C., Higginson, I.J. *et al.* (2004) Evaluation of a short term group intervention for informal carers of patients attending a home palliative care service, *Journal of Pain and Symptom Management*, 27: 396–408.

Henwood, M. (1998) Helping the helpers, *Community Care*, 13–19 August, pp. 22–4.

Higginson, I.J. (1998) Defining the unit of care: who are we supporting and how?, in E. Bruera and R. Portenay (eds) *Topics in Palliative Care*. Oxford: Oxford University Press.

Higginson, I.J. (1999) Palliative and terminal care, *British Medical Journal*, 319: 462–3.

Higginson, I.J. and Priest, P. (1996) Predictors of family anxiety in the weeks before bereavement, *Social Science and Medicine*, 43(11): 1621–5.

Higginson, I.J., Wade, A. and McCarthy, M. (1990) Palliative care: views of patients and their families, *British Medical Journal*, 301: 277–81.

Hileman, J.W. and Lackey, N.R. (1990) Self identified needs of patients with cancer at home and their home caregivers: a descriptive study, *Oncology Nursing Forum*, 17(6): 907–13.

Hinton, J. (1994) Can home care maintain an acceptable quality of life for patients with terminal cancer and their relatives?, *Palliative Medicine*, 8(3): 183–96.

Holicky, R. (1996) Caring for the caregivers: the hidden victims of illness and disability, *Rehabilitation Nursing*, 21(5): 247–52.

Houts, P.S., Rusenas, I., Simmonds, M.A. and Hufford, D.L. (1991) Information needs of families of cancer patients: a literature review and recommendations, *Journal of Cancer Education*, 6(4): 255–61.

Hull, M.M. (1992) Coping strategies of family caregivers in hospice home care, *Oncology Nursing Forum*, 19(8): 1179–87.

Hunt, M. (1991) The identification and provision of care for the terminally ill at home by 'family' members, *Sociology of Health and Illness*, 13: 375–95.

Johnson, I.S., Cockburn, M. and Pegler, J. (1988) The Marie Curie/St Luke's relative support scheme: a home care service for relatives of the terminally ill, *Journal of Advanced Nursing*, 13: 565–70.

Koffman, J. and Higginson, I.J. (2001) Accounts of carers' satisfaction with health care at the end of life: a comparison of first generation black Caribbeans and white patients with advanced disease, *Palliative Medicine*, 15(4): 337–45.

Koffman, J. and Higginson, I.J. (2002) Religious faith and support at the end of life: a comparison of first generation black Caribbean and white populations, *Palliative Medicine*, 16(6): 540–1.

Kristjanson, L., Nikoletti, S., Porcock, D. *et al.* (1998) Congruence between patients' and family caregivers' perceptions of symptom distress in patients with terminal cancer, *Journal of Palliative Care*, 14(3): 24–32.

Lobchuck, M.M. and Kristjanson, L. (1997) Perceptions of symptom distress in lung cancer patients. II: Behavioral assessment by primary family caregivers, *Journal of Pain and Symptom Management*, 14(3): 147–56.

Longman, A.J., Atwood, J.R., Sherman, J.B., Benedict, J. and Shang, T.C. (1992) Care needs of home-based cancer patients and their caregivers: quantitative findings, *Cancer Nursing*, 15(3): 182–90.

McMillan, S.C. (1996) Quality of life of primary care givers of hospice patients with cancer, *Cancer Practice*, 4(4): 191–8.

Miaskowski, C., Zimmer, E.F., Barrett, K.M., Dibble, S.L. and Walhagen, M. (1997) Differences in patients' and family caregivers' perceptions of the pain experience influence patient and caregiver outcomes, *Pain*, 72: 217–26.

Molleman, E., Pruyn, J. and van Knippenberg, A. (1986) Social comparison processes among cancer patients, *British Journal of Social Psychology*, 25: 1–13.

Neale, B. (1991) *Informal Palliative Care: A Review of Research on Needs, Standards and Service Evaluation.* Sheffield: Trent Palliative Care Centre.

Neale, B. and Clark, D. (1992) Informal care of people with cancer: a review of research on needs and services, *Journal of Cancer Care*, 1(193): 198.

Northouse, L.L. and Peters-Golden, H. (1993) Cancer and the family: strategies to assist spouses, *Seminars in Oncology Nursing*, 9(2): 74–82.

Office for National Statistics (2002) http://www.statistics.gov.uk/downloads/theme_health/DH1_34_2001/DH1_34_2001.pdf (accessed July 2004).

Payne, S. and Ellis-Hill, C. (2001) The future: interventions and conceptual issues, in *Chronic and Terminal Illness: New Perspectives on Caring and Carers*, Oxford: Oxford University Press.

Payne, S., Smith, P. and Dean, S. (1999) Identifying the concerns of informal carers in palliative care, *Palliative Medicine*, 13: 37–44.

Payne, S., Large, S., Jarrett, N. and Turner, P. (2000) Written information given to patients and families by palliative care units: a national survey, *The Lancet*, 355: 1792.

Powazki, R.D. and Walsh, D. (2001) Acute care palliative medicine: psychosocial assessment of patients and primary caregivers, *Palliative Medicine*, 13: 367–74.

Rabins, P.V., Fitting, M.D., Eastham, J. and Fetting, J. (1990) The emotional impact of caring for the chronically ill, *Psychosomatics*, 31(3): 331–6.

Randall, T. (1993) Spouses of the chronically ill help each other cope, *Journal of the American Medical Association*, 269: 2486.

Rhodes, P. and Shaw, S. (1999) Informal care and terminal illness, *Health and Social Care in the Community*, 7(1): 39–50.

Schulz, R. and Quittner, A.L. (1998) Caregiving for children and adults with chronic conditions: introduction to the special issue, *Health Psychology*, 17(2): 107–11.

Seale, C. (1989) What happens in hospices: a review of research evidence, *Social Science and Medicine*, 28(6): 551–9.

Seale, C. and Cartwright, A. (1994) *The Year Before Death*. Aldershot: Avebury.

Siegel, K. (1990) Psychosocial oncology research, *Social Work Health Care*, Special issue, *Research Issues in Health Care Social Work*, 15: 21–43.

Slaby, A.E. (1988) Cancer's impact on caregivers, *Advances in Psychosomatic Medicine*, 18: 135–53.

Steele, R.G. and Fitch, M.I. (1996) Needs of family caregivers of patients receiving home hospice care for cancer, *Oncology Nursing Forum*, 23(5): 823–8.

Thorpe, G. (1993) Enabling more dying people to die at home, *British Medical Journal*, 307: 915–18.

Toseland, R.W., Rossiter, C.M. and Labrecque, M.S. (1989) The effectiveness of peer-led and professionally led groups to support family caregivers, *Gerontologist*, 29(4): 465–83.

Toseland, R.W., Blanchard, C.G. and McCallion, P. (1995) A problem solving intervention for caregivers of cancer patients, *Social Science and Medicine*, 40(4): 517–28.

Townsend, J., Frank, A.O., Fermont, D. *et al.* (1990) Terminal cancer care and patients' preferences for place of death: a prospective study, *British Medical Journal*, 301: 415–17.

Willert, M.G., Beckwith, B.E., Holm, J. and Beckwith, S.K. (1995) A preliminary study of the impact of terminal illness on spouses: social support and coping strategies, *The Hospice Journal*, 10(4): 35–49.

World Health Organization (2002) *National Cancer Control Programmes: Policies and Managerial Guidelines*, 2nd edn. Geneva: World Health Organization.

Yeager, K.A., Miaskowski, C., Dibble, S.L. and Wallhagen, M. (1995) Differences in pain knowledge and perception of the pain experience between outpatients with cancer and their family caregivers, *Oncology Nursing Forum*, 22(8): 1235–41.

Young, E., Seale, C. and Bury, M. (1998) It's not like family going is it? Negotiating friendship boundaries towards the end of life, *Mortality*, 3(1): 27–42.

11 | Groupwork in palliative care

Pam Firth

> Groupwork is a deep, rich resource that can be applied to meet many
> different needs in a wide range of settings.
>
> (Manor 2000b: XIV)

This chapter focuses on the variety of methods of group interventions used in the provision of palliative care. Changes in groupwork theories and models are examined briefly and the current state of research discussed. The chapter concludes by looking at the practice issues of running groups for adults and children, illustrating ideas with examples from my own work.

All of us experience groups as we grow and develop, since they are fundamental to human society. For most of us, the human family is our first experience of a group. As we grow up, we move through nursery, playgroup, school and then on to become part of a variety of voluntary groups, such as football teams, Brownies, Scouts and, later, work teams. Groups are hugely significant to us and we know innately when a group is working well or badly. We have experience of joining, leaving and group endings. All these experiences influence our participation in current groups.

In Chapter 2 of this book, Phyllis Silverman traces bereavement theories throughout the last century, linking them to psychological, social and political influences which were then current. Groupwork ideas reflect similar transitions, from the individual in the group, to concepts which have developed from social construction and systemic thinking.

As with the early ideas about bereavement and loss experienced by individuals, groupworkers, group analysts and writers came predominantly from the field of psychoanalysis. The conceptual basis for groupwork is the result of the early knowledge of group dynamics, gained by people such as Bion (1961), Foulkes (1975) and Yalom (1970). This is evident today when discussing such issues as leadership, task and group themes. Bion (1961) has been particularly influential with his ideas about unconscious processes which operate in small groups. He emphasized the way in which the group needs to defend against anxiety. His work highlights the power of the groupwork process, the skill needed to facilitate, and the need for ongoing supervision for leaders of groups.

Levine (1979) reflected the influence of ego psychology with his emphasis on group development, mirroring the development of a maturing individual. All theorists agree that groups go through stages. Manor (2000a), whose model has been heavily influenced by systems theory, is critical of Levine's work. Manor suggests that, in social work practice, most groups do not aim for full emotional growth. He reviewed accounts of groups described in current groupwork journals and found that few aimed to achieve the full course of emotional growth described by Erickson (1965) and used by Levine.

Stages, moods and themes

The idea of stages, moods and themes is accepted by most groupwork writers as being a central part of group life and a way of examining the process.

Four decades ago, Tuckman described his now famous model of sequential stages: 'Forming, Norming, Storming and Performing' (Tuckman 1965). This widely used model has its limitations and is vulnerable to oversimplification if used to examine all group processes in a wide variety of groups.

Doel and Sawdon (1999) describe their Group Work Project in which 66 learners participated by bringing their groups for supervision, scrutiny and evaluation. They concluded that there are clear phases in work with different groups but the phases reflect the aims and tasks of the group. This is particularly evident in experiential groups favoured by counselling training organizations such as Westminster Pastoral Foundation in the UK. My own experience with experiential groups indicates that group material is most likely to be influenced by the current preoccupation raised in the previous lecture of the course.

The benefits which group members gain come from the interactions between group members. Manor (2000a) uses a stage model which centres on communication and feedback. His eight-stage model of communication is shown in Figure 11.1 and can be seen to be focusing on interactive processes. He points out the group's tendency to try to hold on to a steady state (homeostasis) using a systemic theory. In other words, family groups and other groups develop interactive patterns which become resistant to change.

Figure 11.1 The full communication cycle.
(*Source*: Manor 2000a: 85, figure 2.9. Reproduced by permission of the author)

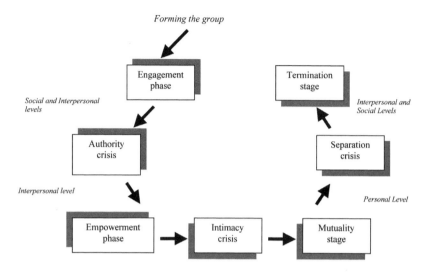

A brief look at systems and systemic thinking

We, as individuals, belong simultaneously to many systems, from our families upwards. Systemic thinking allows us to understand the numerous influences on us and the way in which we try to maintain our boundaries, mobilize change and clarify our moral values in the various groups we belong to. The theory is particularly helpful in enabling us to see the relationships between parts (the members) and the whole (the group) (Thompson 1999: 52; Manor 2000a).

Systems theory emphasizes the point that any system, whether family, group or institution, is particularly fragile at times of transition, for example entrances and exits of members. Some groups have crises as they move between stages (Manor 2000a). For example, a group for bereaved people might have more critical issues to deal with during the Separation Crisis and Termination stage.

Stock Whitaker (1995) also uses ideas from systems theory when she talks about group norms and belief systems. Development of group norms are important and have a regulatory function. The use of norms means that group members do not have to continually go over the rules. Belief systems develop in groups; they are a way of seeing the world and act as a filter. Clearly, group belief systems can be unhelpful and limiting, just as family belief systems can hinder change. In both cases it is important to understand where these systems have come from. Thoughts, ideas and behaviour are often governed by belief systems.

> Two experiential groups met in separate rooms at the same time each week in a counselling centre. The groups held firm beliefs about each other. Group 1 saw themselves as being the sad group; group 2 also felt group 1 was a sad group and tried to develop a belief that their group was strong and happy. Group 1 reflected this and felt their beliefs were true and accurate when they saw group 2 leave relaxed and happy. The two group leaders felt the power of these beliefs but worked with each group and a balance of sadness and happiness was achieved, which reflected more accurately the state of each group at that time.

Thompson (1999: 20) writes that, 'as a group becomes established it begins the process of defining its own reality and forming an opinion as to what sort of group it is and how it compares with the other groups around'.

Each member of a group comes with their own personality, with a personal history and with emotional needs, which they look, to some extent, to satisfy within the group. Observing members, particularly in small groups, it is common to see them playing certain roles, seeking out relationships, which give satisfactory responses. Behaviour is also governed by the feelings that group members have about the group as a whole, as previously discussed. Dissatisfaction with a group can be expressed more easily in the unstructured group but, nonetheless, even in groups with a formal structure, the needs and tensions which individuals bring to a group are always there. Groups need to be able to compromise between the needs of the group members and the task of the group. Defining a task or tasks is one of the most important aspects of groupwork, which raises the issue of group leadership or facilitation.

To summarize:

• Groups are a source of social identity – who we are and what we are worth.
• There is a constant tension in group life between its task and socio-emotional aspects.
• Group dynamics are frequently governed by comparison processes within and without (Brown 2000).

Group leadership

As we consider group leadership, it is important to tackle the issue of group therapy versus groupwork. Is there a difference? Manor (2000a: 36) provides the following helpful definitions:

Group work addresses people's interpersonal and social situations. Group psychotherapy tends to focus on members' internal worlds: the intra-personal processes which give rise to positive symptoms.

The richness of practice is in finding a way of working which suits the situation. The needs of the group members, the task and the setting they find themselves in, will often dictate the way of working. This will also determine the mandate any leader is given. Most people will have had experience of situations where a leader may think they have permission to do one thing but the group wants something else. Unless this is clarified and worked on by the leader and group members, the group will either be paralysed or disintegrate. It is the responsibility of the group leader to clarify the purpose and task of the group.

A social work lecturer ran a weekly discussion group for social work students focusing on their work with their clients. The group consisted of eight students, many of whom were having severe financial problems as they moved into the final year of the course. The discussion became increasingly focused on the financial worries of their clients, to the detriment of other aspects of their clients' problems. The lecturer was forced to examine his role, which was as an educationalist not as a groupworker. His task was to educate not to help solve the problems of his students. By clarifying this, another place was found for the students to find help with their own concerns.

The boxed example demonstrates how easy it is to drift from the task or to assume that the task is clear to all and a mandate given to work in a certain way. New members joining any group will also require the group leader to redefine the task. A further complication is that there is always an educational aspect of the role of group leaders. Most learning for groups follows open-ended questions from the leader, rather than assertions. At times in any group this questioning approach can cause problems, particularly when the group wants certainty. In discussing group leadership, the importance of power and responsibility is emerging.

The group leader's power often comes from their position in the organization and, because they have made the decision about structure and membership, they have the capacity to influence situations within the group. Because of this, members can easily make assumptions about the group leader's power and the way they will exercise it. Here we can see the possibility of early family experiences about power and responsibility surfacing in the group.

Stock Whitaker (1995) introduces the idea of 'stance'. This recognizes the position of the group leader as different from that of the members. The idea is similar to professional distance, referred to in psychotherapy and counselling (Gray 1995). It includes distance and closeness, self-disclosure and level of participation. As with individual work, the group leader works hard to establish a working alliance with the group. Stock Whitaker (1995: 385) describes the working alliance thus:

> The conductors of the group and the members stand together and together face the task of finding ways to tackle issues and/or engage in activities likely to lead to benefit.

A wider systemic view of the working alliance includes also the formal and informal systems involved. This has been developed by Pinsof (1994) and applied to social work practice by Manor (2000c). However, as Stock Whitaker (1995) points out, this does not mean that conflict never occurs between the leader and the group. Conflicts need to be faced, worked on and handled within the safety of the group. A common dynamic is for the group members to talk about a group difficulty outside the group but not to bring it to group meetings. This splitting off is likely when anxieties in the group are high, but it needs to be brought to the group and integrated into the group process. The group leader needs to enable this to happen and face the possible anger of the group. A leader who is not comfortable with conflict severely restricts the group's capacity to learn and grow in confidence.

Firth (2000), while discussing work with staff groups in hospices, describes the difficulty for hospice staff who continually work with high levels of physical and emotional pain and their need for staff support. She points out that staff groups in hospices can use denial, denigration, splitting, projection and idealization to cope with the feelings generated when having such intense experiences with individuals and families on a daily basis. These key psychoanalytical concepts are present in all groups, but if they are understood, linked and discussed safely, they can lead to group members having more realistic expectations of themselves.

Group leaders need to enjoy working with groups. They need to be genuine, respectful, reliable and to take their role seriously, engaging in regular review and supervision. Most group members know if the leader is competent, enjoys the work and is interested in the task.

Self-help groups

So far, the assumption has been made that groups need leaders, but what about self-help groups in palliative care? Urben (1997) comments that most self-help groups in palliative care are run by and for members and have little or no help from professionals. She points out that most research on groups in palliative care is carried out on those facilitated by professionals, usually nurses or social workers, and there has been very little research into self-help groups. Her paper acknowledges, however, that most self-help groups would welcome support from health care professionals.

Breast Cancer Care is supporting the development of training programmes for group facilitators in the UK, working with self-help support groups for women with secondary breast cancer. McLeod (1999) suggests that a key development of the self-help support groups in Breast Cancer Care is that the contribution of facilitators is seen as vitally important.

In my work providing consultation to a group of bereaved parents running a monthly support group, the main issues for those who convened the group, but who did not see themselves as leaders, concerned boundaries and their feelings of entrapment. One person had been bereaved eight years previously. She and her husband wanted to leave the group but felt the group, which was quite fragile, would collapse and leave some newly bereaved parents abandoned. One could see the bind that this couple were in. They felt guilty about setting any limits about when they would leave the group. They gave out their home telephone number and were frequently called late in the evening or at weekends when group members were particularly desperate to talk.

The commonest and most widely available self-help groups are those for the bereaved. Cruse Bereavement Care, The Way Foundation and Compassionate Friends are UK organizations which were founded because there was a recognition that those who have had similar experiences would understand. Currer (2001) argues that most bereaved people look for help beyond those who are already known to them. However, all these organizations, while starting with groups, now offer opportunities for one-to-one support. There is also recognition, particularly in Cruse Bereavement Care, that groups should be led by group leaders who have access to supervision and training.

Examples of groupwork in palliative care

Firth (2000) writes that groups can be very effective in returning power and control to people who are particularly vulnerable and that her experience in running groups for patients, carers and the bereaved lead her to believe that the gains for individuals can be immense. In western society, which is now highly organized and mobile, dying and bereavement can be lonely experiences. Smaller families are often disconnected from their extended family and their original community. Firth (2000) maintains that, in patients' groups, the view that dying is a personal, private experience that other people do not want to hear about, can be countered by open discussions.

In searching the literature for examples of groupwork in palliative care, it is clear that writers describe five types of groups: open, closed, supportive/ reflective, psycho-educational, and long-term therapeutic groups. Sometimes they are a combination of these types, for example, a closed therapeutic group or an open supportive/reflective group. In general, by their very nature, psycho-educational groups are closed because the expectation is that members will come along for a set number of sessions. Indeed, it would prevent group members from processing the impact of the material if people kept coming and going. Closed groups can provide a safer setting for people to share important feelings that need time and space to be explored. In her book about providing a therapeutic frame for one-to-one counselling, Gray (1995) talks about the maintenance of confidentiality, provision of a working place free from interruptions, and regular times for sessions. Groupworkers in palliative care often have difficulty in finding suitable rooms and establishing the need for these rooms to be available at the same time each week. The need for easy access is also vital.

Children's groups

The author ran seven, long-term, closed groups for bereaved young people, which were co-led by two leaders (Firth 1998). The model is of an experiential, psychodynamically oriented group, which used its understandings of the maturation of young people, bereavement, and social networks for young people, to help between six and eight young people negotiate their feelings about the death of a parent or sibling. Groups ran for approximately one year, sometimes longer. These groups had no preplanned programme and were not activity-led, in contrast to those described by Stokes et al. (1997) at Winston's Wish, although games, paper, paint, clay and music were available to be used in the session. Each week the group would bring a topic and, with the agreement of others, this would provide a focus. The boxed example describes one group meeting.

Mary, aged 14, described the night her father died at home and her recurrent nightmares about the events she heard and smelt. Other group members scanned their memories. One boy whose father killed himself told of his experience of being sent into another room when he and his mother returned home from school and how they could see through the glass door a fuzzy image of his father slumped over the kitchen table. This boy said he knew instantly that something was wrong because of his mother's face. It was several days before he was told the truth. His mother had referred him to the group because she said it was as if he was frozen. The group members each told the story of the death in words, pictures and then in clay over several sessions. They would return to this theme when breaks were imminent, as suggested by Manor (2000a) and described earlier in this chapter as the Separation Crisis.

More recently, the author has been involved in running closed activity-based groups for bereaved children and their parent or carer. These groups are planned to take place over four Saturday mornings and involve separate groups for children and for adults but also some whole-group activities. The morning sessions end with children, adults and facilitators sharing a picnic lunch. Feedback has been much the same as described by Stokes *et al.* (1997): it was a positive experience and there appeared to be improved communication between family members.

The children attending both types of group described above had been bereaved in a variety of ways. This fact complicates review and research. Many children whose parents die of cancer have had experience of palliative care and will have had the opportunity to both anticipate their parent's death and benefit from interventions by such staff as the hospice nurses, doctors and social workers, who will have been aware of their needs for inclusion and information.

In a unique groupwork experience, facilitated by Chowns *et al.* (2003) and filmed by the children themselves with the aid of an experienced cameraman, a small group of children with sick parents have made a film called 'No, you don't know how we feel'. The children met for several weeks with four adults, having the joint aims of sharing experiences between the children similarly affected, and making a film which would help other people to enter their world. The group, which consisted of children from 6 to 15 years old, used a range of play, artistic and structured games to act as vehicles, allowing free expression. The children made video diaries and filmed themselves taking part in the activities. They presented a moving insight into the worries and stresses of children, where their lives are governed by a parent with a life-threatening illness. The film ends with the children giving advice to teachers, health care professionals and parents, and is an example of giving service users a voice.

Pfeffer *et al.* (2000) looked at the depressive symptoms, social competence and behaviour problems of pre-pubescent children bereaved within 18 months of parental death from cancer or suicide. They compared the children bereaved by cancer with children who survived their parent's suicide and found that the latter had more depressive symptoms. They suggest that children who have had time to anticipate their parent's death can begin the process of grief before their bereavement. Many authors, such as Parkes (1996), have suggested similar findings with adults bereaved by cancer as opposed to a sudden death. It is strange that much of the work preparing children for parental death has, by all accounts, taken place in one-to-one sessions. The groupwork described above could lead to similar groups taking place (Chowns *et al.* 2003). Health care professionals need to be sensitive to the family's way of adjusting, and care needs to be taken not to undermine parental roles. As cancer moves from a more acute to a chronic disease, families need to adapt and change over time, and the longer-term support of children, many of whom become involved in the care of their parents, is something which needs addressing.

Christ (2000: 22) writes about childhood bereavement:

As we have expanded our knowledge base, we have begun to understand that it is not death or even the particular death itself, that may be the most significant factor in the child's ultimate adjustment, but the supports the child receives, most importantly from the surviving parent. More recently we have found that it is not only the death but also the events that precede the death that may pose the most difficult challenge when death can be anticipated.

Christ (2000: 14) says there is compelling evidence that the death of a parent is better understood by a cascade model than by a single event model; for example, 'The death may trigger a cascade of significant life changes that influence the child's psychological development for a life time, as well as immediately'.

Groups for bereaved adults

There has been much more use of groupwork for bereaved adults than for any other client group within palliative care. The need for social groups to help the bereaved take first steps into the community as single people, has long been recognized, particularly by Cruse Bereavement Care. Sometimes, the bereaved are offered short, focused groups as a way of helping them express their grief. Picton *et al.* (2001) studied psycho-educational groups for bereaved people, which ran for eight weeks. They were particularly interested in looking at such issues as timing and the need for the groups. The programme for the eight-week course included information and practical advice. Timing seemed to be variable, and no firm conclusions were reached as to when people should be offered a group experience.

Generally, bereaved people are not offered groupwork as an intervention until several weeks after their bereavement. My own experience of social group involvement suggests that new members find it very hard early on in their bereavement to join a group and can find it isolating and particularly difficult if other members seem to be enjoying themselves. Another commonly reported problem for leaders of social groups is to help members to leave the group. This difficulty probably arises due to such members experiencing leaving the group as a loss that reminds them of the loss that had led them to joining that group. Many groups have contracted membership entitlement, for example a member can belong to the group for two years. One obvious criticism is the generalization about people's unique experience. Helping members to leave the group requires leaders to work with the crisis and to help members to build their own supportive networks.

There appears to be very little written about group psychotherapy for bereaved spouses. Lieberman and Yalom (1992) describe some brief group psychotherapy with bereaved spouses and compared the outcomes with a group who had no intervention. They found that a psychotherapy model designed for bereaved spouses in helping them meet the psychological and social tasks associated with widowhood had no greater impact than the improvement found in the 'no treatment' control group. The researchers concluded that there is little research focused on what kind of intervention would help, when and with what sort of situation. This subject is visited later in the chapter.

Groups for cancer patients

In a randomized controlled trial by Spiegel *et al.* (1981), a group psychotherapy model was tried as a method of psychological treatment for women with metastatic breast cancer. They found that survival rates improved.

Firth (2000) talks about a patient's discussion group for younger cancer patients and the pre-group planning which reflected anxiety by both patients and staff that there should not be too much dwelling on illness, symptoms, death and dying. The group met during term time, and at the start of each term a programme was arranged. The structure and safety were such that it was possible to discuss all the anxiety-ridden topics, and a culture of openness developed.

The groups developed over time; members died and other members joined, but the group continued. Members began to seek other methods of expression: writing, poetry, painting and making clay models. They sought information by inviting speakers to address issues such as body image, complementary therapies and Chinese medicine. Feedback and attendance were positive.

Many members survived a great deal longer than predicted, which confirmed Spiegel et al.'s work (1981). Members felt that they were often socially dead and had little to contribute to family discussions. This was vividly described by a 19-year-old girl dying of leukaemia, who said that the group made her feel she had something to tell her family when she went home.

Eventually this long-term group closed, a decision taken as a result of management change and service review but without seeking the views of the service users. The staff group wanted to retain a groupwork approach in helping, particularly, younger people with cancer, and so, after much planning, started an eight-week psycho-educational programme, which had the aim of helping people live with cancer. The programme included contributions from outside speakers, such as dentists talking about oral health, as well as members of the multi-professional team, for example physiotherapists giving advice about posture and relaxation. Again, this group has changed over time but continues on a regular basis. It is interesting to note that a number of participants subsequently asked for one-to-one counselling. Groupwork should not be seen as a more economical way to provide therapy, but as one of a range of interventions that can help people.

Other writers discuss psycho-educational groups for cancer patients. Trijsburg et al. (1992) looked at 22 studies of psychosocial interventions in controlled trials and found that 19 reported positive outcomes in most interventions. They concluded that adding a session about coping skills or management of stress produced extra benefits. Cunningham et al. (1999) used a large-group format (more than 20 people) to produce a brief programme which had both clinically and statistically favourable results.

Service user groups

Beresford et al. have considered user involvement in Chapter 8 of this book. Most organizers of hospice and specialist palliative care provision are beginning to engage service users as part of their governance. It makes sense to work in groups which in turn can relate to other service user groups, for example site-specific tumour groups. It is important that these groups are led by experienced people, either users or professionals. Bradburn (2003) makes the point that involvement includes all levels of care and it can be one-to-one. However, the concern of this chapter is to focus on groupwork.

A hospice service user group met three times a year. It was facilitated by two hospice staff and the group was an open one. Notices about meetings were advertised in the press, libraries and within the hospice itself. Generally between 12 and 20 people attended, and transport and food was laid on. At first the theme of each meeting was the idealization of the hospice, but gradually, with support, the culture changed and, after a year, more balanced meetings took place with members contributing both plaudits and criticisms. In turn, the hospice management group became more open to the involvement of the group as natural trust and partnership began to be established.

Observing other service user groups in the NHS in the UK, it is easy to see that the lack of care in providing good, safe rooms with appropriate access, food and transport, contributes to many groups gradually declining. Finally, there is the problem of assuring continuity when we involve service users in strategic planning (Firth 2003); but it is not impossible. One hospice had two user groups: one for bereaved relatives and another for patients and carers. Each group had similar agendas and tasks. They also shared the same leader. The patients' group took place more often and there was sharing of information between groups. More regular meetings allowed for the ill members' absence, due to treatment or whatever. Many patients involved in user groups participate with great determination. Facing their own death, they stress the importance of trying to make things better for others. Broughton (2003: 198), writing as a palliative care user, says: 'User involvement is for me translating users' experience into better services.'

Carers' groups

There are many different examples of carers' groups, from drop-in groups, to psycho-educational groups. Social Services departments have a great deal of experience of all these groups. More recently, the needs of young carers have become very apparent, and local authorities in the UK usually provide dedicated workers to run support groups. Many of the children known to health care professionals in palliative care can be classed as young carers, and their needs for support and, above all, recognition should not be forgotten.

Lesson for research

Bottomley (1997) reviewed two decades of findings regarding group interventions with cancer patients and concluded that there were methodological problems in the research. This was echoed by the work of Stokes *et al.* (1997), who raised the key points relating to why, what and how to evaluate childhood bereavement programmes. They recognized the need to introduce qualitative and quantitative research methods into childhood bereavement literature. Other researchers in this field (for example, Rolls and Payne 2003), explain the difficulty of evaluation. Evaluation should stand up to scrutiny, and clinicians need to link theory, research and the evidence base of childhood bereavement programmes (Stokes 2004).

Piper *et al.* (1992) looked at 25 loss groups for patients. They included a controlled clinical trial of the 'treatment' offered and concluded that short-term group interventions could be successful, particularly where they were tailored to the needs of specific types of patients, in other words, where they were more focused and purposeful. This would link to Bottomley's observation that we should look at the value of specific interventions for patients at different stages of their disease, Bottomley (1997).

Currently, bereavement researchers Silverman and Nickman (1996) and Silverman (2000) suggest that bereaved children negotiate and renegotiate their grief across the life cycle. Maybe there is a need to have open-ended childhood bereavement services as children mature. As Stokes (2004) points out, this would involve a great financial commitment but, for many bereaved children and their parents, being able to 'touch base' with people who understand at least some of what they have lost and who know part of their story, is enormously important.

> A 13-year-old girl joined a long-term group for bereaved young people. Her father had been killed when she was 9 years old. She talked about her confusion as a 9-year-old, but at 13 years of age, she felt a great sense of loss and sadness for the future without a father. Later on, she asked to see the group leader when she went away to university and then when she went to work abroad. This involved two sessions, which appeared to be necessary, reflective pauses in the journey. The group leader felt fortunate to be able to provide this continuity.

Training

This last point above raises issues of selection, training and supervision of groupworkers. It is not normally included in the basic training of most health care professionals involved in palliative care, except for social work training and continues to be widely practised by social workers, particularly in mental health and children and family settings. Some of the advanced training for health care professionals includes groupwork as an option; it has much to offer in palliative care. There might also be the requirement that training should include membership of an experiential group. This is a group with no formal agenda but with the task to explore the group process as it happens. Hutten (1996: 255) writing about experiential groups for trainee counsellors says:

Tasks require individuals to take their own authority to perceive and address them. These groups, which consist of many healthcare professionals, help students think on their feet to take initiatives and to co-operate with others.

Conclusion

This chapter has looked at some of the changes in groupwork practice and examined some specific groups. Groupwork is a creative and exciting way of working. Those attending groups know whether the leader enjoys working with them, and is genuine and respectful. This can only be achieved with enthusiasm, training and good supervision.

When an individual is diagnosed with a life-threatening illness, it is not only the individual but also his family that needs, fundamentally, to reorganize, in order to cope with the demands that illness brings. Groups in palliative care can provide space to allow individuals or family members to find some sort of resolution. Effective group leadership can help groups to keep to task and provide safety and structure, while having in mind the way the group relates to other systems.

The importance of staff caring for themselves and being cared for by the organizations for whom they work has also been discussed. The value of groups in providing both support and education for staff is high. Staff members must always take responsibility for their own care and for the work they do, but having a regular space in which to bring concerns is invaluable.

This chapter has emphasized the need for more research which is methodologically sound. Much of our current knowledge is based around the evidence of the experiences of group members. One thing group members can do is to 'vote with their feet' – unsuccessful groups get smaller. We need to ask people why they leave, as well as concentrating on the experiences of those who stay.

The following quotes are from service users of a hospice group set up to support young bereaved adults, and with which I was involved. The quotes underline the value of this group in providing a space where the bereaved individuals gained support, reassurance, acceptance and approval:

I had no family left when my wife died, no children, just a niece. The group gave me a sense of belonging to someone. If I was unwell, members showed their concern. They also knew what I meant when I talked about chemo. I was very anxious about leaving the group.

Group members look out for each other. I realize now my husband has died, that I am no longer the most special person to anyone. The children don't ask me how I am.

The group has helped me take the first steps towards having a social life. I thought I would never be able to leave the house, except to go to the shops or take the children to school. I realize some of the things I thought or dreamt, such as my husband talking to me, are normal – I am not going mad.

Manor (2000a) suggests that, in groups for the bereaved, the mutuality phase, as he calls it, becomes a central experience for members. The above quotes confirm this.

References

Bion, W.R. (1961) *Experiences in Groups and Other Papers.* London: Tavistock.

Bottomley, A. (1997) Where are we now? Evaluation of two decades of group intervention with adults, carers, patients, *Journal of Psychiatry and Mental Health Nursing*, 4: 251–65.

Bradburn, J. (2003) Developments in user organisations, in B. Monroe and D. Oliviere (eds) *Patient Participation in Palliative Care: A Voice for the Voiceless.* Oxford: Oxford University Press.

Broughton, F. (2003) Conclusion: thoughts of palliative care user, in B. Monroe and D. Oliviere (eds) *Patient Participation in Palliative Care: A Voice for the Voiceless.* Oxford: Oxford University Press.

Brown, R. (2000) *Group Processes.* Oxford: Blackwell.

Chowns, G., Jones, A., Bassey, S. and Lunch, N. (2003) 'No you don't know how we feel'. Video available from gillian.chowns@berkshire.nhs.uk.

Christ, G.H. (2000) *Healing Children's Grief, Surviving a Parent's Death for Cancer.* Oxford: Oxford University Press.

Currer, C. (2001) *Responding to Grief: Dying, Bereavement and Social Care.* Basingstoke: Palgrave.

Cunningham, A.J., Edmonds, C.V. and Williams, D. (1999) Delivering a very brief psychoeducational in a large group format, *Psycho-oncology*, 8: 177–82.

Doel, M. and Sawdon, C. (1999) *The Essential Groupworker.* London: Jessica Kingsley.

Erickson, E. (1965) *Childhood and Society,* London: Penguin.

Firth, P.H. (1998) A long-term closed group for young people, in D. Oliviere, R. Hargreaves and B. Monroe (eds) *Good Practice in Palliative Care*, pp. 86–92. Aldershot: Ashgate.

Firth, P.H. (2000) Picking up the pieces: groupwork in palliative care, in O. Manor (ed.) *Ripples.* London: Whiting & Birch.

Firth, P.H. (2003) Multi-professional teamwork, in B. Monroe and D. Oliviere (eds) *Patient Participation in Palliative Care: A Voice for the Voiceless*. Oxford: Oxford University Press.

Foulkes, S.H. (1975) *Group-Analytic Psychotherapy: Methods and Principles*. London: Gordon & Breach.

Gray, A. (1995) *An Introduction to the Therapeutic Frame*. London: Routledge.

Hutten, J.M. (1996) The use of experimental groups in the training of counsellors and psychotherapists, *Psychodynamic Counselling*, 2(2): 247–55.

Levine, B. (1979) *Group Psychotherapy: Practice and Development*. Englewood Cliffs, NJ: Prentice Hall.

Lieberman, M.A. and Yalom, I. (1992) Brief group psychotherapy for the spousally bereaved: a controlled study, *International Journal of Group Psychotherapy*, 42(1): 117–33.

McLeod, E. (1999) Self-help support groups in secondary breast cancer – a new UK initiative, *European Journal of Palliative Care*, 6(3): 103–5.

Manor, O. (2000a) *Choosing a Groupwork Approach: An Inclusive Stance*. London: Jessica Kingsley.

Manor, O. (2000b) *Ripples*. London: Whiting & Birch.

Manor, O. (2000c) The working alliance, in M. Davis (ed.) *The Blackwell Encyclopaedia of Social Work*, pp. 375–6. Oxford: Blackwell.

Parkes, C.M. (1996) *Bereavement: Studies of Grief in Adult Life*, 3rd edn. London: Tavistock.

Pfeffer, C., Karns, D., Siegal, K. and Jiang, H. (2000) Child survivors of parental death from cancer or suicide: depressive and behavioural outcomes, *Psychooncology*, 9: 1–10.

Picton, C., Cooper, B., Close, D. and Tobin, J. (2001) Bereavement support groups: timing of participants and reasons for them, *Omega*, 43(3): 247–58.

Pinsof, W.M. (1994) An integrative systems perspective on the therapeutic alliance, in A.O. Horvath and L.S. Greenberg (eds) *The Working Alliance*, pp. 173–95. New York: John Wiley.

Piper, W., McCallum, M. and Hassan, F. (1992) *Adaptation to Loss*. London: Guilford Press.

Rolls, L. and Payne, S. (2003) Childhood bereavement services: a survey of UK provision, *Palliative Medicine*, 17: 423–32.

Silverman, P.R. (2000) *Never too Young to Know: Death in Children's Lives*. New York: Oxford University Press.

Silverman, P.R. and Nickman, S.L. (1996) Children's construction of their dead parent, in D. Klass, P.R. Silverman and S.L. Nickman (eds) *Continuing Bonds: New Understandings of Grief*. Washington, DC: Taylor & Francis, pp. 73–86.

Spiegel, D., Bloom, J.R. and Yalom, I. (1981) Group support for patients with metastatic breast cancer, *Archives of General Psychiatry*, 38: 527–33.

Stock Whitaker, D. (1995) *Using Groups to Help People*. London: Routledge.

Stokes, J., Wyer, S. and Crossley, D. (1997) The challenge of evaluating a child bereavement programme, *Palliative Medicine*, 11: 179–90.

Stokes, J.A. (2004) *Then, Now and Always*. Cheltenham: Winston's Wish.

Thompson, S. (1999) *The Group Context*. London: Jessica Kingsley.

Trijsburg, R.W., Vankippenberg, F.C. and Rijma, S.E. (1992) Effects of psychological treatment on cancer patients: a critical review, *Psychosomatic Medicine*, 54(4): 489–517.

Tuckman, B.W. (1965) Development sequence in small groups, *Psychological Bulletin*, 4: 274–84.

Urben, E. (1997) Self-help groups in palliative care, *European Journal of Palliative Care*, 4(1): 26–8.

Yalom, I.D. (1970) *The Theory and Practice of Group Psychotherapy*. New York: Basic Books.

12 Cultural perspectives on loss and bereavement

Shirley Firth

How do minority ethnic people living in the UK cope with death and dying, grieve and mourn? And how can we help them? In addition to the losses faced by everyone after a death, these people often have further issues relating to separation from their homeland, poverty, racism, the situation of the extended family, and command of English.

Professionals may know little about different communities, feel bewildered by unfamiliar attitudes and behaviour and be at a loss in knowing how best to help. There is considerable epidemiological and ethnographic research on minority ethnic communities but limited research into death and bereavement, and therefore little information on cross-cultural perspectives on grief and bereavement. Edited books on cultural perspectives on death and bereavement may provide information about religious beliefs and practices in the countries of origin, but properly researched information about how minority ethnic people in the diaspora deal psychologically with grief and bereavement is almost non-existent (Irish *et al.* 1993; Parkes *et al.* 1997; Morgan and Laungani 2002). Writings on transcultural psychology and counselling do not deal with bereavement, but provide useful insights for those supporting the bereaved (cf. Kareem and Littlewood 1992).

This chapter explores minority ethnic perspectives on loss and bereavement, and examines ways in which professionals can understand and help minority ethnic families. Finally, ways of developing and improving good intercultural practice and appropriate services are discussed, with examples of good practice.

Culture and ethnicity

In health care literature, reference to 'minority ethnic groups' is often made from an ethnocentric perspective, referring to the problems *they* create, as if patients from diverse communities were to be identified by difference rather than giving equal value to all traditions. Culture is something we all inherit, telling us how to view and experience the world and how to behave (Helman 1994; Firth 2001). It is dynamic and changes, especially when confronted by different world-views. People settled in communities more readily retain a sense of identity, which may set them apart, risking misunderstandings and prejudice. Subsequent generations may be bicultural, creating stresses, but crisis and death often renew interest in traditional religious beliefs and practices. Religion, a vital aspect of culture, provides meaning and strategies for coping with suffering and death, although secularized westerners may find it hard to grasp its deep psychic and emotional importance.

The term 'ethnicity' includes culture, language and shared ancestry, but is also determined by a person's self-identity. It is often preferred to 'culture' because the latter has been used to pathologize variations in health (Pfeffer and Moynihan 1996: 68). It may be identified with race and visible difference, racializing and labelling the 'other' as inferior and different (Barot 1993). Reference to 'ethnic minorities' implies that they are heterogeneous, yet each 'community' has wide variations of belief, culture, region of origin, and language. 'Cultural pluralism', 'diversity' and 'multiculturalism' are preferable terms.

Identity is also shaped by family structures, gender, socio-economic status and education. Immigrants, especially refugees, experience multiple changes, losses and possibly trauma, which need to be taken into account in any bereavement work. They may lack emotional and social support; a death may represent loss of a way of life. Uprooting 'disrupts the continuity of an individual's concept of selfhood. ... In particular it disrupts the "structures of meaning", defined by Marris as the conceptual organisation of understanding one's surroundings' (Eisenbruch 1984: 298). Citing Parkes (1986), Eisenbruch shows how the familiar or 'assumptive' ways of looking at the world undergo forcible transitions. Older immigrants may find separation from the homeland and family more acute, especially if the body of the deceased is buried there, with no possibility of visiting the grave (Henley and Schott 1999; Gardner 2002).

Family structures

Many minorities belong to 'collectivist societies', in which the individual is seen in terms of a 'relational' or 'familial self' (Fielding *et al.* 1998).

However, families are fragmenting because of social mobility. This affects attitudes to care, decision-making and bereavement. One cannot assume that minority ethnic families can provide support. Many elders, especially African Caribbeans, experience the triple jeopardy of poverty, racism and poor health, and may have no one to care for them (Blakemore and Boneham 1993).

Interpersonal relationships vary between cultures. For example, in some African families, there are several mothers, with grandparents actively raising children too (Kareem 1992). In the traditional Indian extended family, a wife lives with her husband's parents following an arranged marriage. She is expected to bear sons to continue the lineage and to perform post-mortem rites. An intense bond between mother and son develops partly because his birth validates her identity as a mother and a member of her husband's lineage (Kakar 1978). The loss of a son has long-term economic and social implications if he is the 'old-age pension' and guarantor of care throughout old age.

The emotional bond between marital partners of an arranged marriage may only develop later in life (Kakar 1978). Women acquiring validation by marriage lose it when the husband dies. Hindu widows are considered permanently impure and unlucky, and may be isolated by the husband's family and the community (Firth 1999). The life-long parent–child relationship, maintained by the family's authority structure, may make the loss of a parent profoundly disorientating (Kakar 1978), and the child may 'assume a set of social obligations as prescribed by his ethnic group' (Eisenbruch 1984: 325), identifying more strongly with the beliefs of the parent and culture.

Cross-cultural perspectives on bereavement

It is important to examine how different cultural groups cope with loss and deal with the emotions elicited by death. Do people *express* grief differently, or do they *feel* and experience it differently? Grief is an emotion arising in response to loss; mourning is the way this is expressed, in culturally determined ways; and bereavement is both the state of experiencing grief and the period of time following the death (Parkes and Weiss 1983).

Some sociologists and anthropologists argue that grief is not universal, but socially constructed, in other words that society determines not just how we should behave but also what we actually feel (Radcliffe-Brown 1964; Durkheim 1965; Seale 1998; Walter 1999), while psychologists tend to see a fundamental experience of grief, which may be expressed in different ways according to cultural expectations. Like Eisenbruch (1984), Stroebe and Schut also suggest that there is empirical evidence from biological studies that there are similar emotions of grief in all human beings, which 'provide the fundamental background from which cultural variations should be viewed' (Stroebe and Schut 1998: 7). However, Field *et al.* stress the importance of an interactionist approach allowing for the influence of social contexts, placing 'particular emphasis on communication and meaning and how these affect the experiences of (dying) patients, their relatives and others close to them, and those caring for them' (Field *et al.* 1997: 23).

The theories of stages (Kübler-Ross 1969; Raphael 1984) and tasks (Worden 1991) have been useful tools, if not used prescriptively, for understanding how the bereaved 'work' through the loss, by accepting it, experiencing the pain and adjusting to a newly ordered environment. However, assumptions of universality have been criticized as ethnocentric, whereas in some circumstances and cultures, repression of emotions and memories may be adaptive. We cannot rely on western ideas about 'normal' or 'pathological' grief. Stroebe and Schut (1998) propose a dual process model of grieving, in which at times there is an orientation towards loss, 'letting go of the past', and at other times an orientation towards restoration, remaining with, or keeping hold of, the deceased. This allows for cultural variations, such as the reconstruction of the deceased as an ancestor, who remains in a symbiotic relationship with the living; this is common in Hindu, Chinese and African societies. Walter (1999) also recognizes the importance of creating a place for the dead by talking, locating them in a societal context, and acknowledging the validity of people's experiences of the presence of the dead without reducing them to 'hallucinations'.

'Grief', 'depression' and 'anxiety' are particularly western ways of categorizing and understanding emotional and somatic conditions. English words such as 'guilt' may have different connotations for a white Christian and a Hindu, particularly in the light of concepts such as *karma* and *kismat* (fate). In my research into British Hindu approaches to death (Firth 1997), I found many similar patterns to classic western ones describing numbness, denial, anger and so on, but with some significant differences. First, many informants reported outbursts of violent emotion, not because of expectations but because of the lack of emotional constraints common in British society. Expectations that people should weep publicly during condolence visits and at funerals, were at variance with religious teaching (see below), and some younger Hindus found this difficult. Secondly, while many informants expressed anger against medical staff, there are such deep-seated taboos about expressing anger against a husband, older brother or parent, that no one reported feelings of anger towards these relatives. Finally, while most people found a new meaning and purpose in life, many older widows internalized traditional social attitudes that they were unlucky and impure to the extent that they did not join in social functions at all, spending their lives in prayer for their husbands (Firth 1997, 1999).

Expressing feelings

Emotional reactions may seem extreme in some cultures, but the repression of feelings in others is quite normal. In the Muslim cultures of Egypt and Bali there are contrasting expectations as to how grief should be expressed – overtly in Egypt and controlled and contained in Bali. In Bali, 'suffering was seen as contagious, and detrimental to all ... because expressing one's sadness threatens the well-being of all: the self, the other, and the soul of the dead' (Wiken 1988: 456). Hindus, similarly, see inappropriate emotions as holding the soul back, the consequence of which is that the ghost of the deceased hangs around and harms the living. While they allow space for weeping, tears at an inappropriate time create a river for the soul to cross, and too much attachment impedes its progress (Firth 1997).

As a contrast, in Egypt the response of women to the death of a child is 'to scream, yell, beat their breasts, collapse in each others' arms and be quite beyond themselves for days, even weeks on end', while mothers are expected to remain speechless and listless for weeks (Wiken 1988: 452).

Balinese mothers, including Hindus and Buddhists, cry a little, but try to restrain their grief, suggesting it is the culture and other variables such as social rank, age and gender, rather than the religion which determines behaviour. Japanese, Chinese and Vietnamese may also be reluctant to express emotion, as feelings are private. The ideal is to remain calm and controlled (Boyle 1998).

Depression in the bereaved may not be recognized or acknowledged. Krause (1989) showed that the 'generalized hopelessness' which characterizes depressive disorders in London women would not be regarded as abnormal among Hindu, Muslim and Buddhist women; 'hopelessness' is an aspect of life which can only be overcome on the path to salvation. Widows from many cultures lose status and respectability and may become symbols of bad luck, so are particularly vulnerable (Firth 1999).

Mourning

Mourning is a culturally accepted period of time set in a ritual framework of purposeful activity, which legitimizes social withdrawal and the expression of grief. In established groups there is support following a death, reinforcing bonds between family and caste, clan or community members who provide food and sit with the bereaved, exemplified by the seven days of the Jewish Shiva. Hindus and Sikhs withdraw for ten and more days. Religious readings, homilies and shared narratives about other bereavements place the death in a context of universal experience, reminding the mourners that the death is God's will, and the whole process is in His hands, providing a structural, verbal and conceptual framework within which everyone can express all the many dimensions of their grief, ... the whole process of ... [giving regrets] gives both the immediately bereaved and their entire kinship network an opportunity to review and comment on the fullness of the deceased person's life.

(Ballard, personal communication, in Firth 1997: 154)

These comments are set within a 'framework of meaning by constant reference to the inscrutable powers of the Ultimate'. Life has a purpose, and the deceased has manifestly fulfilled this. Narratives about death perform an important function in maintaining and passing on the tradition, as a source of inspiration and meaning, and as a way of retaining the deceased as a member of the family (Ballard, in Firth 1997).

Cognitive aspects of bereavement and finding meaning

Currer (2001) recognizes that grieving is in part about the meanings which people attribute to life and death. 'It is perhaps only surprising that some theoreticians insist upon the universality of the emotional processes of grief, in the face of apparently contradictory beliefs about the implications of dying (total extinction or the gateway to something better)' (Currer 2001: 55). Concepts of death are affected by radically different views as to its meaning; they may be fearful, with views of hell, or reassuring, with promises of liberation, heaven or rebirth. Models of a good death give meaning to dying. For South Asians, this is in the sacred space of home, with the family around to say farewell and hear last words. Prayers and rituals before death, especially helping the dying person to focus on God, give immense satisfaction, helping the bereaved to know that they have fulfilled their sacred obligations (Firth 1997; Gardner 2002). Some other groups, such as Chinese or Africans, may feel death in hospital is more appropriate.

In cultures believing in survival, it is also important to know that the deceased person has moved on. Many Hindus take comfort from the belief that their deceased relative is reborn, sometimes in the same family, or is 'with God', who is in charge of the cycle of birth and death. The current division between religion and spirituality in much nursing literature does disservice to many religious people, often implying that spirituality is for westerners and religion is for people of other faiths, ignoring centuries of wisdom and insight (Gilliat-Ray 2003). Bereaved people may still have existential and spiritual questions of meaning, and seek metaphysical answers, which may be harder to explore outside their own cultural setting.

Ballard observes that the phrase, 'It is God's will', said by Hindus, Sikhs and Muslims alike to explain suffering, illness and death, is not an expression of fatalism (personal communication, Firth 1997). It is an exploratory remark inviting discussion and dialogue, implying that one will eventually come to see that it is God's will and part of a divine plan, or 'as in the story of Job, part of an educational theodicy' (Dein and Stygall 1997: 296).

Bereavement support

It is evident that many minority ethnic people need bereavement support (Hill and Penso 1995; Spruyt 1999; Netto *et al.* 2001). However, it cannot be assumed that even in closely-knit communities there will be adequate support after the death, and there may be issues which cannot be discussed within the family and social group for reasons of confidentiality (Spruyt 1999; Somerville 2001). If the death was from a stigmatizing disease such as AIDS, there may be no support. Many elderly African Caribbeans are isolated (Blakemore 2000). Older women who have been dependent on their husbands, with restricted access to the outside world, may be thrust into a new world without experience or language skills. They may be isolated and in financial need, requiring help with legal and financial matters (Burrows 1997). Even when there is adequate service provision there may be ignorance of it. Western concepts of counselling may be unfamiliar, particularly as terms like 'bereavement counselling' or 'support' are not readily translatable into other languages. However, once services are made available and publicized, they are utilized (Netto *et al.* 2001; Shoaib and Peel 2003). There may be fears that the service is for white Britons only, or apprehensions about racism, communication and cultural sensitivity. The idea of asking for help and going outside the family for it may seem foreign and bring shame on the person and family (Burrows 1997; Shoaib and Peel 2003). A Sikh woman had two adolescent sons with muscular dystrophy. When the first one died, her husband was so devastated she had to support him emotionally, and did not tell anyone of how she felt unless they asked – which they rarely did – maintaining a serene appearance for both husband and son.

Koffman and Higginson (2001) noted that those African-Caribbean carers who were satisfied with the palliative care services were less likely to experience psychological problems associated with bereavement. The way in which the family member died, the circumstances of the death, experiences of misunderstanding and racism can all complicate bereavement. The most difficult bereavements for my Hindu and Sikh informants were those who were not present at the death and were unable to fulfil their religious obligations (cf. Gardner 2002). Some informants reported a dismal failure by staff to understand religious and emotional needs, which left a bitter taste. Muslims, like Jews, should bury immediately, but unless there is a local Muslim burial plot, and provision for registering the death during weekends and holidays, there can be considerable delays. A post mortem causes immense distress because it is believed that the deceased retains a level of consciousness and can feel pain. Coroners vary as to their sensitivity and willingness to be flexible over the issue. There can be family tensions and disagreements over whether to take a body back to the Indian sub-continent. If a husband's body is returned, the wife may be on her own, unable to make the prescribed visits to the grave (Burrows 1997; Gardner 2002). Hindus and Sikhs, who normally cremate the same day in India, often have to wait a week or more for the funeral in the West. Meanwhile, the structured mourning period has had to shift to before the cremation.

Bicultural individuals and those in mixed marriages may find their grief is complicated if they are pulled in different directions by differing expectations. New conflicts may emerge as the client confronts the life changes ahead.

Case study – Padma

A young Asian woman, 'Padma', was referred to me, following her mother's death. She did not wish to go to an Asian counsellor for confidentiality reasons. A graduate, she had given up an excellent job to look after her dying mother and younger siblings. What emerged was not just her grief for her mother, a deeply loving woman, who had held the family together. Her main difficulties lay in conflict with her father, her inner conflict between her love of and sense of duty to her siblings, reinforced strongly by the local community, who kept assuring her this was her duty, and her longing for an independent life. She realized that she might never be able to marry her Asian fiancé. Her dominating and abusive father insisted she remained at home to care for her siblings, and she did not dare leave them on their own with him, as they were afraid of him.

When someone who 'holds the family together', dies, the consequences can be catastrophic. Padma's cultural and religious background gave her a strong sense of duty and commitment, but her western education offered a wider range of options. She was torn between her own independence, her fear of her father, community pressures and love of her siblings. She did not want advice, but an opportunity to explore the issues confronting her.

Bereavement training

Bereavement support, while requiring training in counselling and listening skills, is not therapy or counselling, although these may be necessary; rather, its purpose is 'to provide a safe place where feelings can be expressed and accepted, and to assure the client that these feelings are normal and that he or she is not going mad' (Walter 1999: 97). The training must enable the counsellor/supporter to grasp the complexities of the cultural context of the bereaved, and some knowledge of intercultural counselling theory and practice is essential. However, much British intercultural counselling theory and training focuses on racial issues, with little reference to bereavement, loss, culture or religion (Kareem and Littlewood 1992). For Taylor-Mohammed this mitigates against training black counsellors, since 'terms such as "intercultural" have often come to be understood in practice, as "How to work with black clients" [which] to a black trainee ... might not be considered as intercultural work at all' (Taylor-Mohammed 2001: 10). While awareness of racial issues, from the perspectives of the client's experience and the supporters' attitudes, is essential, transcultural work also has to take into account the client's background. Different gender roles have to be acknowledged, without western expectations of autonomy and independence affecting judgement of women clients.

Understanding the value of religious practice and beliefs as coping strategies is necessary (Burrows 1997). If supporters/befrienders appear to hold different beliefs and values, clients may feel inhibited about openly expressing fears and emotions (Bahl 1996). However, people without religious beliefs may find it difficult to 'get into the shoes' of those with radically different world-views. Myths about Islam, or negative stereotypes about religion, may engender suspicion and prejudice. Support has, therefore, to be culturally competent, enabling the supporter to lay aside their own cultural expectations and be willing to enter those of the client. The concepts of cultural competence (Leininger 1996) and cultural safety (Ramsden, in Coup 1996) apply to all support contexts, moving beyond practical skills to attitudinal change, which accepts the unique beliefs, values and traditions of different groups, transcending language, ethnicity and culture. They also seek to empower communities themselves to become involved in the development of culturally safe practice in partnership with the majority community (Coup 1996; Oliviere 1999).

Many white workers are anxious about 'not being accepted by the client', of 'being called racist', and of 'not being able to understand', or 'not being understood', or 'being seen as prying' when knowledge of the family's relationships is essential. This may paralyse the visitor, and needs appropriate supervision (Arnold 1992: 156). For Gunaratnam et al. (1998), this involves 'emotional labour', taking informed risks and trusting to intuition. It is important to be honest about our own stereotyping and unconscious racist attitudes. 'Relevant questions about the latter might be "Am I being racist?" and "Am I making inappropriate cultural assumptions about needs and experiences?"' Self-monitoring, as well as welcoming feedback from colleagues, carers and patients, is recommended, with opportunities to share feelings, fears and anxieties in a safe group, thus enabling participants to develop self-awareness and understanding. 'Referential grounding' enables one to see the other person as a similar human being, by finding – or imagining – similar instances in one's own experience, which 'helps to identify ethnic minority people, not as others, but with common needs and experiences' (Gunaratnam *et al.* 1998: 124).

This means avoiding 'shopping lists' of religious or cultural character-istics, finding a balance 'between not overlooking our shared and universal human characteristics and needs, attributing all the client's problems to some "cultural" peculiarity on the one hand, and on the other, neglecting cultural variability with the aim of treating everyone the same' (Arnold 1992: 158; cf. Shoaib and Peel 2003). Arnold suggests we go beyond the external differences and relate as human beings by learning from *inside*, to *know* from real encounters and not just know *about*, getting to know the people we work with *outside* the health care system. Most professionals live in social isolation from minority ethnic groups with no experience of them except in stress situations. We need to develop cultural curiosity, to be willing to explore and get to know the client groups in the area and take delight in the sameness and the stimulus of understanding difference that transcultural relationships brings (Firth 2001).

Education, therefore, needs a much greater commitment than the single afternoon session provided by some services. Netto *et al.* (2001) found that, while mainstream agencies expected counsellors to learn about the rele-vance of cultural and religious issues *from* their clients, black-led organi-sations stressed the importance of understanding the clients' cultural and religious background *before* embarking on counselling. Black counsellors felt that existing training courses were inadequate in preparing counsellors for meeting minority ethnic/black clients' needs. Some of the most useful work on transcultural counselling is written by members of minority communities, both in Britain and the USA (d'Ardenne and Mahtani 1989; Matsumoto 2000; Sue and Sue 2000; Kareem and Littlewood 1992; Lago and Thomson 1996). These throw light on verbal and non-verbal com-munication, race, power and gender issues, and need to be married to studies of bereavement, together with information about the different groups represented in pluralist Britain.

Bereavement services

For multicultural bereavement services to be adequate, training of bereavement supporters/counsellors has to involve both knowledge of cultural issues around death and awareness of different approaches in cultural psychology. Most larger hospices have a bereavement service co-ordinator who will be responsible for recruitment, training and supervision of volunteers, and adherence to national standards. The training needs to include cultural awareness throughout. At Compton Hospice, for example, the training begins with an exploration of participants' own cultural background, challenging their values and attitudes and exploring what 'filters' there may be. It includes respecting and working with diversity, raising awareness on culture and race, sexual orientation, children and adolescents. Specialist trainers add to the programme where possible (Fellowes, personal communication).

Ideally, members of the respective communities will train for bereavement support. However, the concept of voluntary service may not be familiar and may have to be carefully explained. Sikhs have a concept of *seva*, service, a religious obligation to the community, which could be expanded to visiting the ill and bereaved outside the community. The Muslim Bereavement Service in Tower Hamlets, London, was established by the City and East London Bereavement Counselling Service, set up in partnership with the local Bangledeshi community, members of which are serving on the steering committee, and funded for two years by the National Lottery and King's Fund. The service trains Muslim bereavement visitors, with a wider role giving advice when required, making appropriate referrals and acting as advocates. The Sandwell and Dudley Cruse Bereavement Centre in the West Midlands has a freelance African-Caribbean trainer providing cross-cultural bereavement training in the area, including some Asian participants.

Ideally, counsellors/supporters should speak the same language as clients, but there may be reservations about confidentiality. Minority ethnic workers operate in two cultures, with different expectations, needing to be acceptable to both, and be 'defined by clients in terms of a familial relationship' (Fuller 1995: 469). The Sikh advocate at Compton Hospice finds she may be called upon to support Chinese or Caribbean patients and families, who are relieved to find a non-white presence, and she is qualified to do so. However, it cannot be assumed that anyone from a minority community will be able to understand people from other communities, or even their own. Cultural and racial awareness are crucial for anyone in bereavement work, on top of their psychological suitability for working with the bereaved (Netto *et al.* 2001; Shoaib and Peel 2003).

Netto *et al.* (2001) found that South Asian clients initially expected advice, but once they got to know the service, they appreciated being listened to and treated with respect. They also observed that the time boundary was limiting in terms of depth and quality. For some clients the process of familiarization involves preliminary courtesies with offers of drink and food. Some Asian women, who rarely went out, wanted the option of seeing a counsellor at home. Choices regarding the culture, language and gender of the supporter, place to meet, and continuity of care should be available (Burrows 1997; Netto *et al.* 2001). The bereaved may need information about available services, and help with bureaucracy around disposal, including how to register the death, especially during holidays, and when and where to bury or cremate. There may be issues over post mortems. Families may need help over property, wills, housing and future income – how to access help from Social Security and Social Services. Some elders may not be eligible for state help.

Link-workers, advocates and outreach workers have a vital role. Their actual work far exceeds their brief, with the need to help patients, interpret, provide bereavement support and outreach. Acorns Children's Hospice in Birmingham has not only proved outstanding in drawing in children from different minority ethnic groups, but has also provided a service to families with both Asian and African-Caribbean workers (Notta and Warr 1998). A key factor was the appointment of an outreach worker *before* the multicultural service was developed, and who, in addition to running support groups for mothers, provides bereavement support in home visits for as long as necessary. This is not regarded as tokenism, but basic to developing the service (Notta, personal communication).

Conclusion

The variety of types of services suggests the necessity for a more uniform and coherent service throughout the country. Services need to reflect the cultural, racial and ethnic mix of the communities they serve, and they need to be culturally relevant. Recruitment of minority ethnic nurses, social workers, counsellors and bereavement visitors continues to be a priority.

A range of support should be offered, providing choices for those needing it and continuity of support. Publicity in appropriate languages and form (bearing in mind that some potential clients are illiterate), and outreach needs to be developed nationwide (Burrows 1997), with nationally recognized standards of training and qualifications. Policy decisions should acknowledge the diversity of the local communities, guarding against stereotyping and recognizing the clients as unique individuals.

Above all, there needs to be a commitment to diversity throughout the related professions, training and education. Bereavement training has to take into account transcultural studies, from ethnographic and psychological perspectives, and be committed to racial and cultural awareness. While continuing research is essential, the primary issue is to begin investing research findings in creating more appropriate services.

Note

My heartfelt gratitude to Hardev Notta at Acorns Children's Hospice, Allie Fellowes, Dr Pamela Chaudhury and Taj Kaur at Compton Hospice, and the

Muslim chaplain A.K.M. Kamruzzaman and his colleagues at the Birmingham Hospital Trust, for sharing so much with me.

References

Arnold, E. (1992) Intercultural social work, in J. Kareem and R. Littlewood (eds) *Intercultural Therapy: Themes, Interpretation and Practice*, pp. 155–63. Oxford: Blackwell.

Bahl, V. (1996) Cancer and ethnic minorities – the Department of Health's perspective, *British Journal of Cancer*, 74 (Suppl. 29): S2–S10.

Barot, R. (1993) *Religion and Ethnicity: Minorities and Social Change in the Metropolis*. Kampen: Kok Pharos.

Blakemore, K. (2000) Health and social care needs in minority communities: an over-problemetized issue?, *Health and Social Care in the Community*, 8(1): 22–30.

Blakemore, K. and Boneham, M. (1993) *Age, Race and Ethnicity: A Comparative Approach*. Buckingham: Open University Press.

Boyle, D. (1998) The cultural context of dying from cancer, *International Journal of Palliative Nursing*, 2: 70–83.

Burrows, A. (1997) Bereavement, culture and counselling: five Asian perspectives on issues affecting bereaved people of Pakistani descent living in Britain today, and implications for a bereavement counselling service. MA dissertation, Manchester University.

Coup, A. (1996) Cultural safety and culturally congruent care: a comparative analysis of Irhapeti Ramsden's and Madeleine Leininger's educational projects for practice, *Nursing Praxis in New Zealand*, 11(1): 4–11.

Currer, C. (2001) Is grief an illness? Issues of theory in relation to cultural diversity and the grieving process, in J. Hockey, J. Katz and N. Small (eds) *Grief, Mourning and Death Ritual*. Buckingham: Open University Press, pp. 49–60.

d'Ardenne. P. and Mahtani, A. (1989) *Transcultural Counselling in Action*. London: Sage.

Dein, S. and Stygall, J. (1997) Does being religious help or hinder coping with chronic illness? A critical literature review, *Palliative Medicine*, 11: 291–8.

Durkheim, E. (1965) *The Elementary Forms of the Religious Life*. New York: Free Press (first published 1912).

Irish, D.P., Lundquist, F., and Jenkins, V. (eds) (1993) *Ethnic Variations of Dying, Death and Grief: Diversity in Universality*, Washington DC: Taylor & Frances.

Eisenbruch, M. (1984) Cross-cultural aspects of bereavement II: Ethnic and cultural variations in the development of bereavement practices, *Culture, Medicine and Psychiatry*, 8(4): 315–47.

Field, D., Hockey, J. and Small, N. (eds) (1997) *Death, Gender and Ethnicity*. London: Routledge.

Fielding, R., Wong, L. and Ko, L. (1998) Strategies of information disclosure to Chinese cancer patients in an Asian community, *Psycho-social Oncology*, 7: 240–51.

Firth, S. (1997) *Dying, Death and Bereavement in a British Hindu Community*. Leuven: Peeters.

Firth, S. (1999) Hindu widows in Britain: continuity and change, in R. Barot, S. Fenton and H. Bradley (eds) *Ethnicity, Gender, and Social Change*. Basingstoke: Macmillan.

Firth, S. (2001) *Wider Horizons: Care of the Dying in a Multicultural Society*. London: National Council for Hospice and Specialist Palliative Care Services.

Fuller, J. (1995) Challenging old notions of professionalism: how can nurses work with paraprofessional ethnic health workers?, *Journal of Advanced Nursing*, 22: 465–72.

Gardner, K. (2002) *Age, Narrative and Migration: The Life Course and Life Histories of Bangladeshi Elders in London*. Oxford: Berg.

Gilliat-Ray, S. (2003) Nursing, professionalism, and spirituality, *Journal of Contemporary Religion*, 18(3): 335–49.

Gunaratnam, Y., Bremner, I., Pollock. L. and Weir, C. (1998) Anti-discrimination, emotions and professional practice, *European Journal of Palliative Care*, 5(4): 122–4.

Helman, C. (1994) *Culture, Health and Illness*. Oxford: Butterworth-Heinemann.

Henley, A. and Schott, J. (1999) *Culture, Religion and Patient Care in a Multiethnic Society*. London: Age Concern.

Hill, D. and Penso, D. (1995) *Opening Doors: Improving Access to Hospice and Specialist Palliative Care Services by Members of the Black and Ethnic Minority Communities*. London: National Council for Hospice and Specialist Palliative Care Services.

Irish, D.P., Lundquist, F. and Jenkins, V. (eds) (1993) *Ethnic Variations in Dying, Death and Grief: Diversity in Universality*, Washington, DC, Taylor and Francis.

Kakar, S. (1978) *The Inner World: A Psychoanalytic Study of Childhood and Society in India*. Delhi: Oxford University Press.

Kareem, J. (1992) The Nafsyat Intercultural Therapy Centre: ideas and experience in intercultural therapy, in J. Kareem and R. Littlewood (eds) *Intercultural Therapy: Themes, Interpretation and Practice*, pp. 14–37. Oxford: Blackwell.

Kareem, J. and Littlewood, R. (eds) (1992) *Intercultural Therapy: Themes, Interpretations and Practice*. Oxford: Blackwell.

Koffman, J. and Higginson, I. (2001) Accounts of carers' satisfaction with health care at the end of life: a comparison of first generation black Caribbeans and white patients with advanced disease, *Palliative Medicine*, 15(4): 337–45.

Krause, I. (1989) The sinking heart, a Panjabi Communication of Distress, *Social Science Medicine*, 29(4): 563–75.

Kübler-Ross, E. (1969) *On Death and Dying*. London: Tavistock.

Lago, C. and Thompson, J. (1996) *Race, Culture and Counselling*. Buckingham: Open University Press.

Leininger, M. (1996) Response to Cooney Article, 'A comparative analysis of transcultural nursing and cultural safety', *Nursing Praxis in New Zealand*, 22(2): 13–15.

Matsumoto, D. (2000) *Culture and Psychology*. Belmont: Wadsworth.

Morgan, J.D. and Laungani, P. (2002) *Death and Bereavement Around the World*. Vol 1: Major Religious Traditions, Baywood Publishing Co. Inc, NY, Amityville.

Netto, G., Gaag, S. and Thanki, M. (2001) *A Suitable Space: Improving Counselling Services for Asian People*. Bristol: The Policy Press for Joseph Rowntree Foundation.

Notta, H. and Warr, B. (1998) Acorns Children's Hospice, Birmingham, in D.K. Oliviere, R.K. Hargreaves and B. Monroe (eds) *Good Practices in Palliative Care: A Psychosocial Perspective*. Aldershot: Ashgate Arena, pp. 148–50.

Oliviere, D. (1999) Culture and ethnicity in palliative care, *European Journal of Palliative Care*, 6(2): 53–8.

Parkes, C. (1986) *Bereavement: Studies of Grief in Adult Life*. London: Penguin.

Parkes, C. and Weiss, R. (1983) *Recovery from Bereavement*. New York, Basic Books.

Parkes, C.M., Laungani, P. and Young, B. (eds) (1997) *Death and Bereavement Across Cultures*. London: Routledge.

Pfeffer, N, and Moynihan, K. (1996) Ethnicity and health beliefs with respect to cancer: a critical review of methodology, *British Journal of Cancer*, 74, Suppl. XXIX: S66–S72.

Radcliffe-Brown, A. (1964) *The Andaman Islanders*. New York: Free Press.

Raphael, B. (1984) *Anatomy of Bereavement*. London: Unwin Hyman.

Seale, C. (1998) *Constructing Death: The Sociology of Dying and Bereavement*. Cambridge: Cambridge University Press.

Shoaib, K. and Peel, J. (2003) Kashmiri women's perceptions of their emotional and psychological needs, and access to counselling, *Counselling and Psychotherapy Research*, 3(2): 87–94.

Somerville, J. (2001) The experience of informal carers within the Bangladeshi community, *International Journal of Palliative Nursing*, 7(5): 240–7.

Spruyt, O. (1999) Community-based palliative care for Bangladeshi patients in East London: accounts of bereaved carers, *Palliative Medicine*, 13: 119–29.

Stroebe, M. and Schut, M. (1998) Culture and grief, *Bereavement Care*, 17(1): 7–11.

Sue, D. and Sue, D. (2000) *Counselling the Culturally Different*. New York: John Wiley.

Taylor-Mohammed, F. (2001) Follow fashion monkey never drink good soup: black counsellors and the road to inclusion, *Counselling and Psychotherapy Journal*, 12(6): 10–12.

Walter, T. (1999) *On Bereavement*. Buckingham: Open University Press.

Wiken, U. (1988) Bereavement and loss in two Muslim communities: Egypt and Bali compared, *Social Science Medicine*, 27: 451–60.

Worden, J. (1991) *Grief Counselling and Grief Therapy*, 2nd edn. London: Routledge.

13 | Conclusions

Pam Firth, Gill Luff and David Oliviere

Anything that you have, you can lose,
anything you are attached to, you can be separated from,
anything you love can be taken away from you.
Yet, if you really have nothing to lose, you have nothing.

(Kalish 1985: 181)

Loss, change and bereavement

Throughout this book there are examples of research, practice and individual stories from people struggling to understand the meaning of loss. From the First World War of 1914–18 through to the third millennium, experiences and interpretations of bereavement, loss and change have evolved significantly in a global sense. There has been a move from the colossal, but often somewhat concealed, reality of loss, through to the equally devastating but infinitely more public, such as the Space Shuttle Columbia disaster (February 2003), the horrors of 11 September 2001, and of genocides, famines and wars. However, our task has been to look at the current and the particular within today's context: the experiences of individuals, families and small groups, facing life-threatening illness or bereavement. Good practice in palliative care has involved the recognition of the needs of those experiencing loss and change, coupled with the exploration of appropriate ways of supporting them (Sheldon 1997). The authors in this book have examined how people's identities are framed by relationships with others (Silverman, Chapter 2; Machin, Chapter 3; Pam Firth, Chapter 11). The loss of an important relationship is felt to be an attack upon the self. Silverman suggests that grieving involves changes in how we see ourselves but it must also include examining our relationship with the deceased. Altschuler (Chapter 4) makes the point that some life-changing events can be helpful whereas others are more challenging and require much more reorganization of our sense of self.

The creation of stories and talking to people who knew the deceased give mourners a chance to grieve over time and to process their loss (Walter 1999). This includes children who also need to do this as they grow and develop. Self-esteem, security and confidence are eroded when a person – adult or child – is bereaved. The challenge is for society to give people space and time for these important processes and to engage with them in a natural but sensitive way so as not to isolate or dismiss them. The rich mixture of people in our society with different ethnicities but shared common needs and experiences calls for professionals who are culturally competent to hear and react to their stories (Shirley Firth, Chapter 12). There are opportunities for hospice and palliative care services to provide groups for children and adults in which they can share their loss with others (Pam Firth, Chapter 11). Grief is, indeed, an interactional process. The social context of people's lives includes work, religious and cultural customs, and school. In addition to the public and media interest in bereavement support and counselling following trauma, disasters and the increasing threat of terrorism, there is a growing awareness of the need not only to provide death education in schools but also to set up systems which support bereaved schoolchildren (Rowling and Holland 2000; Stokes 2004). Work-based counselling services are increasingly provided by large companies and organizations as part of occupational health services. However, the majority of people do not need counselling, but they do need friends, colleagues and family members who can listen. But how do we encourage people to listen adequately? A basic reminder of the importance of listening comes from Remen (1996: 143):

> I suspect that the most basic and powerful way to connect to another person is to listen. Just listen. Perhaps the most important thing we ever give each other is our attention. And especially if it is given from the heart. When people are talking, there's no need to do anything but receive them. Listen to what they are saying. Care about it. Most times, caring about it is even more important than understanding it.

Most of the authors in this book talk about the multiplicity of change that people have to make when they are seriously ill or bereaved. How much do we know about the complexity of change and its huge impact? Christ (Chapter 7) stresses that we need a deeper understanding of the mechanisms of change, although Parkes' (1993) long-standing interest in change has informed us by describing and defining 'psychosocial transitions' as life-changing events which challenge our assumptive world. Family therapists (McGoldrick and Walsh 1991) talk of changes across the life cycle that relate to the ordinary tasks of families at different stages, and how death and serious illness can be particularly challenging where it occurs 'out of time'.

Western cultures worship young, fit, healthy people. Meanwhile, Altschuler (Chapter 4) talks about how we all have a passport to illness, but it is a passport we shun. Are we prepared for the shifts and changes in society as populations age? Who will care for the increasingly numerous older members of society? What can their contribution be?

> One of the most hurtful misconceptions about the process of ageing is the assumption that at some point in their lives people inevitably stop growing personally. The result is that all too often older people are treated as if they have already stopped living.
>
> (Reoch 1997: 14)

Charmaz (1995) makes a similar point about seriously ill people, who are often regarded as socially dead, by those around them. Hearn (Chapter 9) also highlights aspects of old age, linking it to unequal access to relevant palliative care services, which similarly applies to other disadvantaged groups on the margins of society, such as those with learning disabilities, prisoners and minority ethnic groups.

The National Institute for Clinical Excellence (NICE) guidance on cancer services in England and Wales, underlines the importance of the development and implementation of services that focus both upon bereavement as well as needs generated through the duration of illness (National Institute for Clinical Excellence 2004). But clearly the experience of loss and change is not confined to those who are ill or bereaved. It impacts upon those closest to them, and to those involved with their care, as illustrated by Harding (Chapter 10). Based on UK experiences, Ellis-Hill and Payne (2001) remind us that the partnership model, which acknowledges the rights and needs of carers as proposed by the Carers' National Strategy (Department of Health 1999), should shift and redress the uneven power differential experienced by carers in their dealings with professionals.

Research

Research continues to challenge our assumptions and reminds us not to be dismissive in relation to some former strongly held models and theories. For instance, Stroebe (2002) examines the impact of attachment theory upon contemporary research, focusing upon the seminal works of Bowlby (1969, 1980) and Parkes (1996, 2001). Stroebe's study and collaboration helped to extend theories of attachment to the field of bereavement. She recognized that their contributions were strongly entwined, through their joint work at the Tavistock Clinic, London, but with Bowlby concentrating in the early stages on deprived children, while Parkes focused and enlarged upon the bereaved individual. Stroebe goes on to show how her own model, the dual process model (DPM) of oscillating grief, developed with Schut (Stroebe and Schut 1999), links coherently with attachment theory propositions. These illustrate secure versus insecure types of attachment, making links between current coping mechanisms and earlier experiences. Stroebe (2002: 135) concludes that, 'what we have now is not just a description of the types of coping that are (mal)adaptive but a suggestion as to how these patterns are related to styles of attachment'.

There are salutary reminders that not all commonly held ways of helping bereaved people are supported by research evidence. In their critical examination of the efficacy of grief interventions, Schut *et al.* (2001) revealed some uncomfortable contraindications. They found methodological difficulties in comparison across a wide range of efficacy studies internationally. Nonetheless, non-selective 'blanket' grief interventions were found to be uncertain in their effectiveness, although the results were more promising where children's grief interventions were studied and compared. However, studies that concentrated upon interventions for complicated grief provided modest but positive, long-lasting results. We are reminded that research needs to push out the boundaries of how we listen most effectively to the bereaved: their needs, outcomes and best practices in partnership.

Resilience

Kissane emphasizes that the adaptation following bereavement is associated with personal growth for a sizeable proportion of people and this is identifiable across all phases of the bereavement process. 'Reasoned sense of meaning, self awareness, increased empathy, appreciation of family relationships, independence, reprioritised goals and values, deepened spirituality and increased altruism can all result from positive reappraisal' (Kissane 2003: 1147).

Similar findings emerge from the worldwide research on resilience and how people achieve despite adversity (Bluglass 2003; Oliviere, forthcoming). Resilience, the capacity to do well when faced with difficult circumstances (Vanistandael 2003), has always been evident in those receiving palliative and bereavement care. Even work with complex bereavement situations teaches us much of how people are resilient, despite loss, trauma and devastating change. Traditionally there has been an emphasis on identifying bereavement risk and vulnerability factors rather than strengths and ways of promoting resilience. The Liverpool Children's Project was initiated following the Hillsborough football stadium disaster in 1989, and its objective in providing bereavement support was to increase the capacity of family, friends and communities to support and enhance children's potential for resilience (Barnard *et al.* 1999). It has been demonstrated that resilient children are better equipped to resist stress and adversity, cope with change and uncertainty, and to recover faster and more completely from traumatic events or episodes (Newman and Blackburn 2002). These factors, better understood, may help services to adapt to better meet needs (Rutter 1985; Barnard *et al.* 1999).

The word 'resilience' has come into our present usage from the study of physics, signifying springiness, the ability to re-form after bending, stretching or compression (Bluglass 2003; Vanistandael 2003).The International Resilience Project, which collected data from 30 countries, described resilience as 'a universal capacity which allows a person, group or community to prevent, minimise or overcome damaging effects of adversity' (Newman and Blackburn 2002: 1). Palliative and bereavement care can benefit from considering aspects of resilience and what sustains people in trauma, however important it is to assess risk. Models and frameworks that have helped us understand coping mechanisms in recent times lend themselves to appreciating bereaved people's resilience (Stroebe and Schut 1999; Machin, Chapter 3 in this book).

Research needs to focus on the complexity of interacting processes of vulnerability and resilience, risk and protective factors, in order that we understand further the relationship. As clinicians and practitioners, researchers and policy-makers, we need to go on learning how bereaved people maintain competent functioning despite the emotional, psychological, spiritual and social challenge that is bereavement. We need to continue to become more skilled in harnessing positive coping strategies (Oliviere forthcoming).

Bereaved people are a rich source of dynamic data and the value of the user movement in palliative and bereavement care is increasingly recognized, which has potential for better informed research and practice (Relf 2003). Projects to capture feedback from service users are expanding and build on the record of bereaved parents and others' work in writing their stories and creating new groups and services. In many ways, the individual voice is strong but the collective voice needs to be facilitated more powerfully through forums of all sorts, email contact, ad hoc groupings and other interactive methods of feedback. The voice of service users can make a significant difference to what services are planned and provided. Beresford *et al.* (Chapter 8) emphasize that there is a strong tendency to consider user involvement as additional rather than fundamental. The way forward should be to recognize the user's role at the centre of all policy and service provision.

User involvement taps into the healthy side of people by attempting to balance the patient–professional partnership in a mutual alliance. It is one of many ways of demonstrating the creativity that can result from the experience of loss, change and bereavement. Stunning examples are emerging of users of palliative care contributing to the initiation, planning, development, operation and evaluation of services; and in education, research and publication. At St Christopher's Hospice in London, for example, work is beginning with Listening Days for staff to receive feedback from users 18–24 months post bereavement. This offers users an opportunity to inform professionals of the quality of services from a perspective some distance after the death. In addition, an active Users' Education Advisory Group of patients and carers, chaired by a bereaved carer, samples, monitors and feeds back to ensure the educational courses are patient-centred.

The challenge for bereaved people is to go on integrating their painful life experiences into their present-day lives. We have shown how people *can* do this and how different models of support help and encourage them in this process.

> It is perfectly true, as philosophers say...
> Life can be understood by looking backwards, but they forget to add that it also has to be lived forwards.
> (Kierkegaard 1843, in Bluglass 2003)

References

Barnard, P., Morland, I. and Nagy, J. (1999) *Children, Bereavement and Trauma: Nurturing Resilience*. London: Jessica Kingsley.

Bluglass, K. (2003) *Hidden from the Holocaust: Stories of Resilient Children who Survived and Thrived*. London: Praeger.

Bowlby, J. (1969) *Attachment and Loss. Vol. 1, Attachment*. London: Hogarth Press.

Bowlby, J. (1980) *Attachment and Loss. Vol. 3, Loss: Sadness and Depression*. London: Hogarth Press.

Charmaz, K. (1995) The body, identity and self: adapting to impairment, *Sociological Quarterly*, 36(4): 657–81.

Department of Health (1999) *Carers' National Strategy*, HMSO.

Ellis-Hill, C. and Payne, S. (2001) The future: interventions and conceptual issues, in S. Payne and C. Ellis-Hill (eds) *Chronic and Terminal Illness*. Oxford: Oxford University Press.

Kalish, R. (1985) *Death, Grief and Caring Relationships*, 2nd edn. California: Brooks-Cole.

Kissane, D. (2003) Bereavement, in D. Doyle, G. Hanks, N. Cherney and K. Calman (eds) *Oxford Textbook of Palliative Medicine*, 3rd edn. Oxford: Oxford University Press.

McGoldrick, M. and Walsh, F. (1991) A time to mourn: death and the family life cycle, in F. Walsh and M. McGoldrick (eds) *Living beyond Loss: Death in the Family*. New York: W.W. Norton.

National Institute for Clinical Excellence (2004) *Guidance on Cancer Services:*

Improving Supportive and Palliative Care for Adults with Cancer. London: NICE.

Newman, T. and Blackburn, S. (2002) *Transitions in the Lives of Children and Young People: Resilience Factors.* Edinburgh: Scottish Executive Education Department.

Oliviere, D. (forthcoming) *Resilience and Palliative Care.*

Parkes, C.M. (1993) Bereavement as a psychosocial transition: processes of adaptation to change, in M. Stroebe, W. Stroebe and R. Hansson (eds) *Handbook of Bereavement: Theory, Research and Intervention.* Cambridge: Cambridge University Press.

Parkes, C.M. (1996) *Bereavement: Studies of Grief in Adult Life,* 3rd edn. London: Routledge.

Parkes, C.M. (2001) A historical overview of the scientific study of bereavement, in M. Stroebe, R.O. Hansson, W. Stroebe and H. Schut (eds) *Handbook of Bereavement Research: Consequences, Coping and Care.* Washington, DC: American Psychological Association.

Relf, M. (2003) Bereavement care, in B. Monroe and D. Oliviere (eds) *Patient Participation in Palliative Care: A Voice for the Voiceless.* Oxford: Oxford University Press.

Remen, R. (1996) *Kitchen Table Wisdom: Stories that Heal.* New York: Riverhead Books.

Reoch, R. (1997) *Dying Well: Holistic Guide for the Dying and their Carers.* London: Gaia.

Rowling, L. and Holland, J. (2000) Grief and school communities: the impact of social context, a comparison between Australia and England, *Death Studies,* 24: 35–50.

Rutter, M. (1985) Resilience in the face of adversity: protective factors and resistence to psychiatric disorder, *British Journal of Psychiatry,* 147: 598–611.

Schut, H., Stroebe, S., Van Den Bout, J. and Terheggen, M. (2001) The efficacy of bereavement interventions: determining who benefits, in M. Stroebe, R. Hansson, W. Stroebe and H. Schut (eds) *Handbook of Bereavement Research: Consequences, Coping and Care.* Washington, DC: American Psychological Association.

Sheldon, F. (1997) *Psychosocial Palliative Care: Good Practice in the Care of the Dying and Bereaved.* Cheltenham: Stanley Thornes.

Stokes, J. (2004) *Then, Now and Always.* Gloucester: Winston's Wish and Calouste Gulbenkian Foundation.

Stroebe, M. (2002) Paving the way: from early attachment theory to contemporary bereavement research, *Mortality,* 7(2): 127–38.

Stroebe, M. and Schut, H. (1999) The dual process model of coping with bereavement: rationale and description, *Death Studies,* 23: 197–224.

Vanistandael, S. (2003) Resilience and spirituality. Unpublished paper.

Walter, T. (1999) *On Bereavement.* Buckingham: Open University Press.

Index